MW01518001

"Based on the latest scientific research, John-Tyler Binfet and Elizabeth Kjellstrand Hartwig have produced a unique and important guide to the implementation of canine-assisted interventions in settings ranging from classrooms and retirement facilities to mental health clinics and college campuses. The book is a veritable how-to manual, covering topics such as the selection and training of handlers and dogs, the assessment of dog/handler team effectiveness, and therapy animal welfare. This book is a must-read for anyone involved with animal-assisted intervention programs."

—**Hal Herzog, PhD**, author *of Some We Love, Some We Hate, Some We Eat: Why It's So Hard to Think Straight About Animals*, USA

"Drawing on a wealth of experience, John-Tyler Binfet and Elizabeth Kjellstrand Hartwig provide a comprehensive review of what is known about canine-assisted interventions (CAIs) and give essential information on best practice and how to credential therapy dog teams, ensuring the well-being of the dogs. CAI organizations and those interested in becoming a CAI team must read this book."

—**Anthony L. Podberscek**, editor in chief, *Anthrozoös*, Australia

"*Canine-Assisted Interventions* is an essential guide to all those involved in delivering and researching canine-assisted interventions. It provides evidence-based guidelines for professional practice, building upon current international research evidence and professional practice guides. The combination of up-to-date scientific evidence on canine-assisted intervention and professional experience has led to a sourcebook that every practitioner involved in canine-assisted intervention should use. Canine-assisted intervention practice is growing rapidly around the world, and this book provides a much-needed guide to credentialing teams and ensuring our practice benefits our human clients while ensuring the welfare of the dogs we work with."

—**Jo Williams**, professor of applied developmental psychology, University of Edinburgh, UK

"In *Canine-Assisted Interventions*, John-Tyler Binfet and Elizabeth Kjellstrand Hartwig bring together a groundbreaking, thorough, and detailed guide to the assessment and credentialing of dog and handler teams. This long-overdue resource is a much-needed and indispensable resource for individuals and organizations engaged in the work of animal-assisted interventions. Binfet and Hartwig articulate a clear and thorough evidence-based approach to animal-assisted intervention that will significantly advance this growing field of research and practice."

—**James Gillett**, associate dean of research, McMaster University, Canada

Canine-Assisted Interventions

Covering principles of therapy dog team training, assessment, skills, and ongoing monitoring, *Canine-Assisted Interventions* provides guidance on the most evidence-based methods for therapy dog team welfare, training, and assessment.

The authors offer a linear approach to understanding all aspects of the screening, assessment, and selection of dog/handler teams by exploring the journey of dog therapy teams from assessment of canines and handlers to the importance of ongoing monitoring, recredentialing, and retirement. In addition to reviewing key findings within the field of human-animal interactions, each chapter emphasizes skills on both the human and dog ends of the leash and makes recommendations for research-informed best practices. To support readers, the book culminates with checklists and training resources to serve as a quick reference for readers.

This book will be of great interest for practitioners, in-service professionals, and researchers in the fields of canine-assisted interventions and counseling.

John-Tyler Binfet, PhD, is an associate professor in the Faculty of Education at the University of British Columbia, where he is the director of the Building Academic Retention through K9s program. (B.A.R.K.; barkubc.ca).

Elizabeth Kjellstrand Hartwig, PhD, LPC-S, LMFT, RPT-S, is an associate professor in the Professional Counseling Program at Texas State University. She is the founder and director of the Texas State University Animal-Assisted Counseling Academy (aac-academy.clas.txstate.edu).

Canine-Assisted Interventions

A Comprehensive Guide to Credentialing
Therapy Dog Teams

John-Tyler Binfet and
Elizabeth Kjellstrand Hartwig

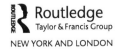
Routledge
Taylor & Francis Group

NEW YORK AND LONDON

First published 2020
by Routledge
52 Vanderbilt Avenue, New York, NY 10017

and by Routledge
2 Park Square, Milton Park, Abingdon, Oxon, OX14 4RN

Routledge is an imprint of the Taylor & Francis Group, an informa business

Library of Congress Cataloguing-in-Publication Data
A catalog record for this book has been requested

ISBN: 978-1-138-33830-2 (hbk)
ISBN: 978-1-138-33831-9 (pbk)
ISBN: 978-0-429-43605-5 (ebk)

Typeset in Goudy
by Apex CoVantage, LLC

John-Tyler Binfet:
This book is dedicated to Frances Binfet, both a rescue and a rescuer.

Elizabeth Kjellstrand Hartwig:
This book is dedicated to my parents, Bill and Leslie Kjellstrand, who have supported my love for animals in many ways, and to my therapy dog, Ruggles, for teaching me the true purpose of counseling.

Contents

Figures

Tables

Boxes

Meet the Authors

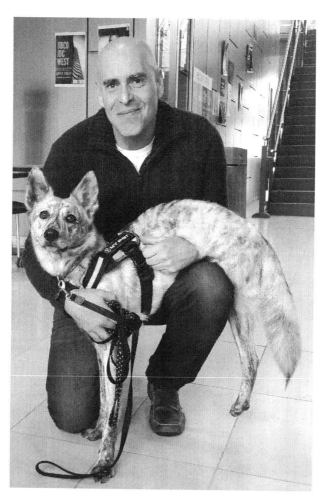

John-Tyler Binfet is an associate professor in the Faculty of Education at the University of British Columbia (UBC), Okanagan campus. His research explores prosocial behavior in children and adolescents and the effects of canine-assisted interventions on college student well-being. Dr. Binfet is the lead author of the School Kindness Scale and his research on kindness explores how students understand and enact kindness within school contexts. Since 2014, Dr. Binfet has been a board member of the Social and Emotional Learning Special Interest Group for the American Educational Research Association and is an editorial board member for the *Journal of Childhood Studies, Anthrozoös,* and the *Human-Animal Interaction Bulletin.* Dr. Binfet is the founder and director of UBC's dog therapy program B.A.R.K. (Building Academic Retention Through K9s). His research explores the effects of therapy dogs on college students' perceptions of stress, homesickness, and connectedness to one another. Dr. Binfet's research on canine-assisted interventions has been published in *Anthrozoös, Society & Animals,* the *Journal of Veterinary Behavior,* and the *Journal of Mental Health.*

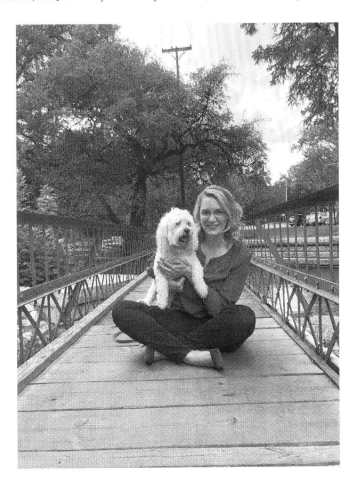

Elizabeth Kjellstrand Hartwig is an associate professor in the Professional Counseling Program at Texas State University, where she teaches animal-assisted counseling, play therapy, and marriage and family therapy courses. She is the founder and director of the Texas State University

Animal-Assisted Counseling (AAC) Academy, a professional training program that promotes the human-animal bond through the study and practice of animal-assisted counseling. Dr. Hartwig pioneered the first involvement of therapy dogs on the Texas State University campus. She has facilitated studies on animal-assisted counseling, developmental assets in youths, and resiliency factors in single mothers. Dr. Hartwig is a past president of the Texas Association for Play Therapy (TAPT). In 2017, she received the TAPT Nancy Guillory Award for Outstanding Service in Play Therapy. She has presented on animal-assisted counseling and play therapy at regional, national, and international conferences, including presentations in the United Kingdom, France, and Australia. Dr. Hartwig has a private practice in New Braunfels, Texas, called Pawsitive Family Counseling, LLC, where she partners with her therapy dog, Ruggles.

1   Introduction

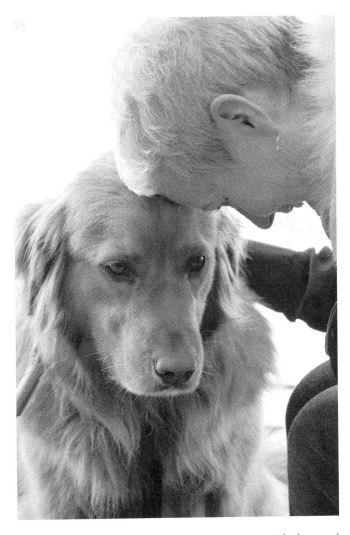

Figure 1.1 An employee at a local police precinct connects with therapy dog Nava from UBC's B.A.R.K. program.

Whether you're a community volunteer, program director, potential client to a session, or researcher, you've picked up this book because of your interest in canine-assisted interventions (CAIs, or what you might call "canine-assisted therapy") and the potential it has to support a variety of well-being outcomes. Our aim in writing this book is to provide evidence-based, current information on all aspects of working with therapy dogs—from screening and assessment procedures through credentialing and retirement. In addition to reviewing key findings within the field of human-animal interactions (HAIs), each chapter showcases innovative work in the field and makes recommendations for research-informed best practices.

As professionals working in the field of HAI, we've seen firsthand the benefits that therapy dogs provide to a variety of clients in a range of contexts. Our work has been fueled by clients who, when gently petting a therapy dog, look up with tear-filled eyes and say, "Thank you." As researchers investigating the effects of CAI, we understand the importance of designing studies and using methodologies that contribute to the evidence attesting to the power of therapy dogs to effect positive change in people's lives—to boost well-being. We understand the importance of training protocols for handlers and practitioners, of the duration of interventions, and of both qualitative and quantitative research designs that help discover findings to advance the field. One aim in writing this book is to enhance practice, and within each chapter, we'll illustrate, in applied ways, the steps involved in supporting and enacting CAIs. In short, we want to encourage the advancement of CAIs through sharing evidence-based findings to inform best practices.

The Surge in Popularity of CAIs

The field of CAIs is certainly dynamic, and the early founders of this approach to supporting human well-being would undoubtedly be surprised at its current popularity and growth. Whereas historically we might have seen one therapy dog and handler volunteer to support the well-being of a senior citizen in a retirement care facility, we now see therapy dogs in programs supporting a wide array of clients. This includes but is not limited to CAI teams volunteering in the following contexts (see Table 1.1).

We also see dogs working alongside professionals in the following contexts (see Table 1.2).

The rapid expansion that now sees therapy dogs placed in a variety of public settings has raised concerns among researchers and practitioners alike, as the research attesting to the benefits of this approach hasn't caught up to the surge in popularity. That is, you have organizations implementing CAIs in an expansive assortment of contexts to support a wide variety of clients, yet the research supporting these practices is lagging. In fact, and at the time of our writing this book, in reviewing the list just presented illustrating the varied contexts within which we find CAIs implemented, a review of the extant psychological, anthrozoological, and veterinary research reveals peer-reviewed findings attesting to the benefits of therapy dogs within less than half of these contexts.

Table 1.1 CAIs Across Volunteer Contexts

Setting	Clients	Target Outcome(s)	Applied Example	Peer-Reviewed Evidence
Airport	Travelers	Reduce stress and anxiety	www.fodors.com/news/photos/12-north-american-airports-where-you-can-pet-a-therapy-dog	No evidence found
College campus	College students	Reduce stress, anxiety, and homesickness	www.huffingtonpost.ca/entry/therapy-dogs-ease-stress-college-students_us_5b84d6f3e4b0511db3d10b98	Barker, Barker, McCain, & Schubert (2016) Binfet (2017) Binfet, Passmore, Cebry, Struik, and McKay (2018) Grajfoner, Harte, Potter, and McGuigan (2017) Ward-Griffin et al. (2018)
Crisis center	Crime victims	Reassure and comfort crime victims	www.pghcitypaper.com/pittsburgh/a-new-program-pairing-child-abuse-victims-with-dogs-helps-with-healing/Content?oid=3061085	No evidence found
Dental office	Pediatric dental patients	Reduce anxiety during visit	www.ada.org/en/publications/ada-news/2015-archive/may/pediatric-dentist-shares-dental-therapy-dog-success-story	Nammalwar & Rangeeth (2018) Schwartz & Patronek (2002)
Elementary school	Children	Improve reading skills and confidence	www.tdi-dog.org/OurPrograms.aspx?Page=Children+Reading+to+Dogs	Connell, Tepper, Landry, and Bennett (in press) Kirnan, Siminerio, and Wong (2016) Kirnan, Ventresco, and Gardner (2017) Le Roux, Swartz, and Swart (2014) Linder, Mueller, Gibbs, Alper, and Freeman (2018)

Table 1.1 (Continued)

Setting	Clients	Target Outcome(s)	Applied Example	Peer-Reviewed Evidence
Fire station	Firefighters	Reduce stress	www.orlandosentinel.com/news/orange/os-ne-ocfr-first-therapy-dog-20190211-story.html	No evidence found
Funeral home	Grieving families	Reduce grief	www.therapydogs.com/therapy-dogs-offer-comfort-funeral-services/	No evidence found
Homeless shelter	Homeless individuals	Reduce tension among residents within the facility	https://globalnews.ca/news/3997811/montreal-homeless-shelter-uses-therapy-dog-to-bring-comfort/	No evidence found
Hospital	Inpatients and outpatients	Reduce stress, facilitate pain management, and improve hemodynamics	www.usnews.com/news/beststates/oklahoma/articles/2019-02-04/therapy-dogs-bring-smiles-pain-relief-to-lawton-hospital www.cbc.ca/news/health/pet-therapy-dogs-1.4952949	Chubak et al. (2017) Cooley & Barker (2018) Harper, Dong, Thornhill, Wright, & Ready (2015) Kline, Fisher, Pettit, Linville, and Beck (2019)
Law office	Legal clients	Assist lawyers with mediation between clients	www.petguide.com/blog/dog/therapy-dogs-helping-lawyers-mediate-divorces/	No evidence found
Long-term care facility	Elderly residents	Improve mood and cognitive functioning and reduce depression	www.westhawaiitoday.com/2019/01/23/hawaii-news/here-comes-riley-therapy-dog-brings-comfort-and-smiles-to-life-care-center-of-kona/	Lutwack-Bloom, Wijewickrama & Smith (2005) Thodberg et al. (2016)
Medical settings	Medical residents/nursing students	Reduce stress	www.studyinternational.com/news/college-introduces-therapy-dogs-reduce-medical-students-stress/	Crossman, Kazdin, and Knudson (2015) Delgado, Toukonen, and Wheeler (2018) Norton, Funaro, & Rojiani (2018)
Military base	Service members	Facilitate openness to communicate personal health issues	www.af.mil/News/Article-Display/Article/1756663/army-therapy-dog-visits-maintenance-airmen/	No evidence found

Table 1.1 (Continued)

Police department/precinct	Police officers	Reduce stress and boost well-being within the precinct	www.rcmp-grc.gc.ca/en/gazette/k9-comfort?gz	Binfet, Draper, & Green (in press)
Public library	Children	Foster reading interest and motivation, and improve literacy skills	www.kltv.com/2019/02/14/paws-reading-program-success-longview-library/	Hughes (2002) For a review see Newlin (2003)
Public tragedies/ disaster relief	Victims and mourners	Provide comfort to victims and mourners after a public tragedy	www.orlandosentinel.com/news/pulse-orlando-nightclub-shooting/os-care-dog-pulse-night-club-20160617-story.html www.ctvnews.ca/canada/therapy-dogs-providing-comfort-after-toronto-van-attack-1.3907322	No evidence found For a review see Shubert (2012)
Recovery center	Clients struggling with addiction	Help in addiction recovery	www.rehabcenter.net/therapy-dogs-helpful-in-addiction-rehabilitation/	Contalbrigo et al. (2017) Kelly and Cozzolino (2015) Wesley, Minatrea, and Watson (2009)
Safe house/ recovery center	Women and children	Provide comfort	www.comoxvalleyrecord.com/community/therapy-dog-has-2000-service-hours-to-credit/	No evidence found

Table 1.2 CAIs Across Professional Contexts

Setting	Clients	Target Outcome	Applied Example	Peer-Reviewed Evidence
Audiology clinic	All ages	Reduce anxiety during visit	https://canadianaudio logy.ca/ member-spotlight-kathleen-jones-exploring-the-benefits-of-animal-assisted-therapy/	No evidence found
Physical therapy	All ages	Promote physical mobility	www.vetstreet.com/ our-pet-experts/the-amazing-ways-dogs-are-helping-kids-with-physical-therapy	Elmaci and Cevizci (2015)
Speech therapy	Children with speech-language challenges	Enhance communication	https://leader.pubs. asha.org/doi/ 10.1044/leader. MIW2.11022006.34 https://medibulletin. com/kids-in-speech-therapy-respond-better-with-a-dog-around/	Machová et al. (2018)
Counseling	All ages	Reduce stress or symptoms of depression/ improve mental health	www.socialworktoday. com/ archive/031513p6. shtml https://people.com/ pets/pet-therapy-eating-disorders-soul-paws/	Calvo et al. (2017) Dietz, Davis, and Pennings (2012) Hartwig (2017) Lange, Cox, Bernert, and Jenkins (2006/2007) Prothmann et al. (2005) Prothmann, Bienert, and Ettrich (2006)

This surge in implementation is the opposite of the typical or standard research trajectory that sees a small intervention piloted and, should initial findings be favorable, the pilot program tested in further studies, including the gold-standard, randomized controlled trial, which is a complex methodological approach in which participants are randomly assigned to treatment and control conditions. Should favorable findings, such as benefits to human well-being, be found after further empirical investigation, then, and only then, would a program be launched and implemented in applied ways.

Here, in our current landscape of CAIs, we have a few well-run studies that indicate this modality, this means of supporting human well-being, shows promise; however, studies certainly have not been conducted in all of the contexts and with all of the client populations in which we currently find CAIs implemented. What is further troubling is that the conditions of an experimental study, run by highly trained researchers, in which we see therapy dogs participate, do not mirror the conditions found in applied, real-world settings that see therapy dogs interacting with varied members of the public. Thus, therapy dogs who work well under research conditions may not participate as enthusiastically or support clients to the same extent within loosely monitored public programs under the guidance of informally trained personnel. Further, we have researchers who, under carefully controlled experimental conditions, report that therapy dogs do not experience elevated stress during sessions as reflected by biomarker and observational data, yet the average context within which community-based programs are enacted sees therapy dogs working in markedly different conditions than those found in experimental studies. Caution must be exercised when interpreting research findings for applied settings, especially during a time of rapid growth that sees new iterations of CAIs all the time.

What's Propelling the Interest in CAIs?

We suspect that there are at least four forces driving this surge in, and expansion of, CAIs: First, there is the strong desire by the public to spend time with dogs. In our fast-paced, technologically driven world, finding contact with nature, with living beings other than humans, can be a challenge. Theory supports this interpretation, and Wilson's (1984) biophilia hypothesis argues we are drawn to life and lifelike organisms. Thus, when opportunities present themselves that afford members of the public to spend time with dogs, they jump at the chance as it fulfills a basic need to connect with nature.

Second, social media plays a role in spreading anecdotal evidence claiming that spending time with therapy dogs is beneficial. A college student who posts a selfie of himself and an on-campus therapy dog with the caption "This is the reason I'm still on campus" helps convince all his followers that spending time with therapy dogs yields positive benefits to well-being. This creates a culture of supporters who are convinced, without any corresponding scientific evidence, that spending time with therapy dogs boosts student retention rates.

Third, CAIs have seen a spike in popularity across contexts and with varied client populations because it is a surprisingly low-cost intervention. Fueled predominantly by volunteer resources, programs operate in communities with little overhead and no facilities and run on the goodwill of volunteers and passionate program directors.

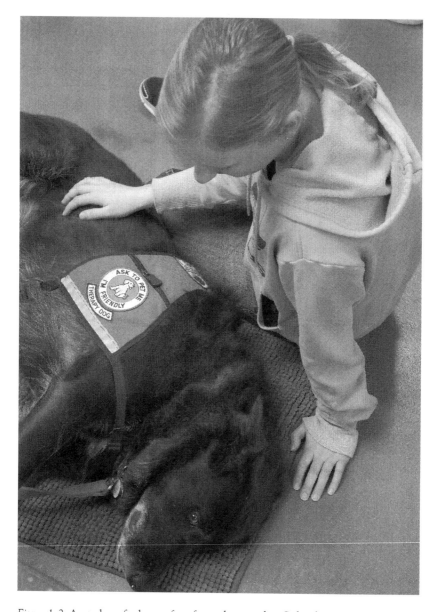

Figure 1.2 A student finds comfort from therapy dog Siska from UBC's B.A.R.K.
program.

Last, the popularity of CAIs is fueled, in part, by the intrinsic and extrinsic gratification received by volunteer handlers and practitioners. Helping
others by sharing one's dog and witnessing the impact of this sharing on the
well-being of clients is intrinsically gratifying for handlers. The appreciation

expressed by clients around how meaningful the interaction is serves to reinforce and provide extrinsic feedback to handlers. Together, the intrinsic and extrinsic feedback experienced by handlers keeps them partnering with therapy dogs, often enthusiastically, in CAIs and thus keeps CAI organizations afloat and thriving.

Challenges in the Field of CAIs

Two challenges are evident in the field of CAI: First, there is ample ambiguity in the terms used to refer to all things CAI. Second, there is variability in just how the designation of "therapy dog" is bestowed on or allocated to a CAI team. These variabilities can be perplexing both for prospective CAI teams and for the public, and our hope in writing this book is that we both clarify and streamline language around CAI and clarify the screening, training, and assessment required for a dog and handler to be credentialed as a CAI team.

As we'll establish throughout this book, there is variability in virtually all aspects of CAIs. This variability can be confusing for researchers and practitioners alike, and an examination of this variability is in order as we lay a foundation for readers in understanding all things CAI.

Variability in Background and Training

First, there is variability in the background and training of the individuals who start and run CAI organizations. You might see and could have individuals with a keen interest in dogs and a few obedience classes under their belts running a program, all the way up to folks with PhDs or veterinary medical degrees and advanced training in the field of HAIs running organizations. The background, experience, and training of organization personnel are important, as this knowledge base influences decision-making around all the aspects that make an organization run—from the type of assessments used to identify CAI teams, to how canine welfare is protected during sessions out in the field. What training should the director of a CAI organization have? Where might one obtain training in CAIs?

Variability in Language

Variability is also found in the language used to describe CAIs. The field is rife with parallel terms and acronyms, with stakeholders using different and nuanced language to essentially describe the same approach or protocol. Even when national-level organizations attempt to clarify terminology, it seems new acronyms and terms crop up. This variability serves to muddy the waters in advancing understanding of, and work in, the field of CAI.

In addition to streamlining CAI-related language, we argue in this book that there is a need to clarify and strengthen the screening, training, and assessment practices used to identify CAI teams. We highlight later in this

Table 1.3 Terminology Related to CAIs

Term	Definition/Understanding
Canine-assisted intervention (CAI)	The bringing together of credentialed CAI teams and members of the public in a specified setting with the purpose of enhancing human well-being. May be delivered individually with one CAI team and one client or group administered with several CAI teams supporting multiple clients.
CAI organization	A group whose mission is to provide public access to CAI teams.
CAI program	Developed under the supervision of a CAI organization, a series of CAI sessions within a specific context designed to support specified clients.
Handler	Within the context of this book, the owner/guardian of the therapy dog, typically a volunteer community member within an organization.
Practitioner	A term used to describe a professional who works with a canine as part of her or his professional responsibilities. Might include a counselor, social worker, physical therapist, or occupational therapist. Requires advanced training.
Therapy dog	A dog assessed for behavior, skills, and disposition who works under the guidance of a handler or practitioner and who participates in interactions to support the social, emotional, and/or physical development of clients.
CAI team	A term to describe a therapy dog and handler or practitioner who work collaboratively within CAIs as volunteers for an organization or as professional practitioners.
CAI client/ recipient/ visitor/patient	An individual in a community or professional setting who interacts with a CAI team in an effort to promote wellness.
CAI team assessment	The process through which a prospective CAI team is assessed to determine suitability for credentialing as a CAI team.
CAI team credentialing	The process of screening, training, and assessing the skills of a CAI team to work in a volunteer or professional capacity on behalf of a CAI organization.

chapter the importance of handler and practitioner screening and training, as this has been an oft-overlooked aspect of the credentialing process. For the purposes of our writing and in an effort to streamline vocabulary within the field, we operationally define the following terms for use here (see Table 1.3).

CAI Terminology

These terms streamline and reduce variability in the descriptions of stakeholders and actions commonplace in the CAI field. To be sure our distinctions are clear for readers, therapy dogs are not facility dogs, courthouse facility dogs, psychiatric service dogs, emotional support animals, service dogs, or working dogs. To reiterate, therapy dogs are dogs who live with volunteer handlers or professional practitioners ("owners," if you will, or "guardians") who have been screened, trained, and assessed by personnel from a CAI organization for participation in community-based programs or professional practices that support the well-being of clients. The credentialing of a CAI team provides no public access rights, and the team is limited to the scope of work for which the team has been assigned. In Chapter 3, we discuss, in depth, the duties and responsibilities of both dogs and handlers working within CAIs on behalf of an organization.

One key dimension of the work undertaken by therapy dogs is the scope and breadth of clients they support across varied contexts (See Figure 1.3 here).

As Figure 1.3 illustrates, therapy dogs may work in a variety of different contexts and with varied members of the public. Prior to delving into the temperament and skills required of handlers, it's important to discuss the question, What draws pet dog owners to want to share their dogs with the public? Certainly, the phrasing "therapy dog" can be misleading, as this is a broad term that describes more generally "canine visitation" rather than the delivery of therapy in the traditional sense. Certainly, there has been ample confusion on the part of the public in understanding the role of therapy dogs and differentiating their role from service dogs or emotional support dogs. This is evidenced by owners bringing therapy dogs or even pet dogs into restaurants or public spaces reserved for working service dogs. Airline companies and the public alike, however, are increasingly aware of the rights and privileges accorded to certified service dogs, and owners trying to bend the rules around public access can find themselves quickly admonished. There is even discussion underfoot to prosecute members of the public who try to pass pet dogs as service dogs. Titled "Criminalizing Fake Service Dogs: Helping or Hurting Legitimate Handlers?" this publication by Tiffany Lee (2017) published in *Animal Law* provides an overview of the legal ramifications of fraudulent service dog practices.

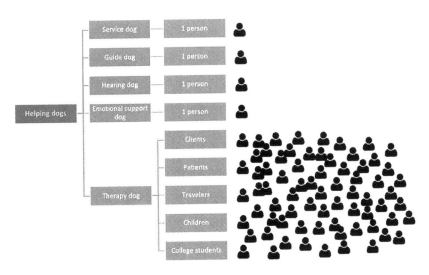

Figure 1.3 Illustration of the number and variety of clients supported by therapy dogs.

As an illustration of the importance of this topic, take the experience of Hugh Saunderson and his guide dog, Niobe, who encountered an aggressive "service" dog during an outing to their local shopping mall. Profiled in a Canadian Broadcasting Corporation piece titled "Fake Service Dogs a Menace for Legitimate Owners, Businesses Alike" (Burke, 2018), the story of Mr. Saunderson, who is legally blind, depicts the tale of an encounter with an aggressive and poorly managed "service" dog while out in public. With the increase in owners masquerading pet dogs as service dogs, individuals reliant on service dogs find themselves and their dogs at increasing risk and their dogs' abilities to support their independence compromised.

Though Mr. Saunderson's experience at his local mall illustrates a dramatic threat to his service dog's ability to provide him support, there are countless small, daily intrusions that compromise service dogs' abilities to support their handlers. A military veteran on a recent outing to a local hardware store with his PTSD service dog relayed the story of people approaching his dog and moving the dog's service vest, the vest with clearly labeled patches indicating the dog is working and not to be pet, in order to give his dog a scratch or hug. Further complicating these interactions, this veteran tells of the public asking, "How do I get a dog like this? I want one!" Considering this service dog provides support to a veteran to counter the psychological effects of having served in the Canadian military, the insensitivity of such questions is especially problematic.

The increase in pet dog owners purchasing service vests online for their dogs to gain access to public space reflects, perhaps, the desire owners have to spend time with their dogs. Once relinquished to the backyard, dogs now hold coveted spots in their owners' lives. In response to, and as a reflection of, this shift, a burgeoning and lucrative pet care industry has arisen that sees canine day care facilities in urban centers, canine spas, canine-themed events at local pubs in which owners and their dogs are welcome, and a plethora of fashion items and accessories for dogs. In short, the role of dogs has changed, with dogs very much positioned as family members, and it is not surprising, although highly misguided, that we find owners wishing to extend their appreciation of their dogs to broader, public spheres by having them masquerade as service dogs.

One avenue through which owners may both spend time with their dogs and be in a public setting is through participation in a CAI as part of a CAI organization. Such participation affords pet owners opportunities to share their dogs with others through structured programs that support a variety of clients' well-being. Next, we'll explore the variability in the process of identifying a therapy dog and handler for work as a CAI team.

Variability in CAI Team Credentialing

Variability in Screening, Training, and Assessment

Related to the training of CAI organization personnel is the variability we find in the type and scope of training and assessments done to determine that the team is well suited for CAIs. As we'll establish throughout this book, we see too little scrutiny of prospective CAI teams before determining a team is of sound character, disposition, and skills worthy of a CAI team designation. As Linder and colleagues (2018) reported, one third of the canine programs in their study relied uniquely on the Canine Good Citizen (AKC, 2019) test to determine whether a CAI team was a good fit for CAI work. Undoubtedly, even the folks who developed the Canine Good Citizen test would agree that this test was not crafted for the purpose of identifying therapy dogs. As we argue in Chapter 5, it may play a role in screening potential CAI teams, but on its own, it has limited applicability as a sole indicator for CAI work. CAI organization personnel seeking to screen potential CAI teams might consider requiring the Canine Good Citizen certificate as part of their screening process, as this would be an indication of the handler's commitment to attending CAI training and completing the CAI credentialing process.

Variability in Programs and Settings

As the popularity of spending time with therapy dogs has grown and as the research attesting to the benefits of therapy dogs has emerged, the demand for CAI teams in varying contexts has increased. We now routinely see therapy dogs participating in programs in a variety of settings to support the well-being of a variety of clients. Throughout this book we provide illustrations of the various contexts within which CAI teams are found, as well as the nuanced training required of these teams for work within these varied settings. One issue arising from the varied contexts and clients that we see therapy dogs working in and supporting is that the training and assessment practices to identify CAI teams for work within these contexts do not reflect just what is required of teams within these settings. Thus, a generic credentialing of a CAI team does not guarantee that the team is capable of the work required within the specialized context (more on this in Chapter 8). A CAI team who is credentialed to work with one health-impaired, geriatric client in a retirement facility for seniors could potentially be ill prepared to meet the demands of clients seeking to reduce their stress in a busy airport.

Variability in the Scientific Evidence Supporting CAIs

Despite the popularity of research examining the effects of therapy dogs on an array of human well-being outcomes, caution within the scientific community has been raised regarding the rigor of research done in this burgeoning field. Herzog (2011, 2014), Marino (2012), and more recently Crossman (2017), and Crossman, Kazdin, Matijczak, Kitt, and Santos (2018) have written about the need for more rigorous research and argue for caution in proclaiming causality in animal assisted–themed research (i.e., that therapy dogs cause boosts to human well-being). Specifically, these authors argue that research rigor can be derived from the use of random assignment to treatment and control conditions and that studies need to be done that isolate just what it is about spending time with therapy animals that produces positive benefits (e.g., tactile touch). The topic of research rigor is picked up again in our last chapter where we propose guidelines for researchers and argue for research standards when CAI teams participate in studies investigating the effects of CAIs.

Clarifying the CAI Team Credentialing Process

In an effort to reduce some of the variability we see across all aspects of CAIs and to both support and align the efforts of people working to identify strong CAI teams, we propose the following credentialing process (see Figure 1.4).

Integral to this model is sequencing, and our model sees a potential CAI team pass through a series of phases or protocols that allow them to showcase their best skills and dispositions while allowing a CAI organization ample and sufficient opportunities to assess these skills and dispositions vis-à-vis their needs, mission or vision, and goals for community programming, professional placements, or research. Figure 1.4 informs the sequence of our subsequent chapters, and in the following section, we provide a brief overview of what to expect as you read each of the chapters that follow.

Overview of Chapters

This book will begin with an overview of CAIs. Chapter 2 will situate CAIs within the broader context of HAIs. We'll also clarify the theories or mechanisms of CAI that contribute to positive outcomes and answer the question, How does it work exactly? Chapter 3 will then explore the foundational skills, behaviors, and dispositions required by a CAI team in order to become credentialed by an organization. Chapter 4 will provide an overview of considerations around safeguarding CAI client and canine well-being. This includes an examination of both the factors contributing to elevated stress in therapy

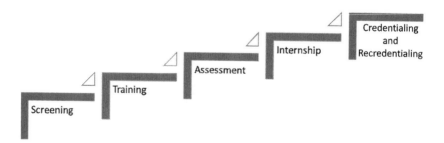

Figure 1.4 CAI team credentialing process.

dogs and the indicators of stress in dogs. As the field of CAI advances so, too, have the calls to ensure that therapy dogs, who oftentimes work in busy settings with stressed clients, are looked after. Could the very intervention designed to promote well-being in humans be distressing for therapy dogs? Chapter 5 will explore best practices in training CAI teams. This includes a description of prerequisite and CAI team skills needed for assessment and credentialing. Chapter 6 will introduce and provide an overview of canine-assisted counseling, an area where therapy dogs might find themselves working alongside mental health practitioners. Chapter 7 will provide an overview of comprehensive approaches to CAI assessment. Oftentimes the canine is the focus of assessments, but the handler plays a critical role in the delivery of programming and the attainment of desired outcomes, and Chapter 7 will help readers understand and identify key aspects contributing to strong handler performance. In Chapter 8, we'll provide an overview of assessment considerations for specialized contexts. Should a therapy dog working in an elementary school's reading program be assessed differently than a dog working with a health-impaired client in a quiet hospital setting? Chapter 9 will explore how best to ensure dogs and handlers continue to be well suited to the work they're assigned to do. How might dogs and handlers be monitored once they're credentialed by a CAI organization? Our last chapter, Chapter 10, provides an overview of new and anticipated developments in the field. In this chapter, readers will find an accreditation checklist for CAI organizations to help monitor their ability to implement and deliver gold-standard practices and programs.

Conclusion

As researchers working in the field of CAIs, we have a responsibility to share findings that help advance knowledge. As practitioners, we want to ensure that programs run in the best interest of all stakeholders, including those at the heart of the therapeutic process: the therapy dogs themselves. We offer this book as a platform to inform both the science and the practice of all dimensions of CAIs and trust it will inspire your work in the rewarding field of CAIs.

References

American Kennel Club (2019). *Canine good citizen*. Retrieved from www.akc.org/products-services/training-programs/canine-good-citizen/

Barker, S. B., Barker, R. T., McCain, N. L., & Schubert, C. M. (2016). A randomized cross-over exploratory study of the effect of visiting therapy dogs on college student stress before final exams. *Anthrozoös*, 29(1), 35–46. doi: 10.1080/08927936.2015.1069988.

Binfet, J. T. (2017). The effects of group-administered canine therapy on first-year university students' well-being: A randomized controlled trial. *Anthrozoos*, 30, 397–414.

Binfet, J. T., Draper, Z. A., & Green, F. L. L. (in press). Stress reduction in law enforcement officers and staff through a canine-assisted intervention. *Human-Animal Interaction Bulletin*.

Binfet, J. T., Passmore, H. A., Cebry, A., Struik, K., & McKay, C. (2018). Reducing university students' stress through a drop-in canine-therapy program. *Journal of Mental Health, 3*, 197–204. doi: 10.1080/09638237.2017.1417551.

Burke, A. (2018, March 9). Fake service dogs a menace for legitimate owners, businesses alike. *Canadian Broadcasting News*. Retrieved November 4, 2018, from www.cbc.ca/news/canada/ottawa/ontario-hotels-fake-service-animal-scam-1.4567432

Calvo, P., Pairet, S., Vila, M., Losada, J., Bowen, J., Cirac, R., . . ., & Fatjó, J. (2017). Dog assisted therapy for teenagers with emotional and behavioural issues: A multi-centre study. *European Psychiatry, 41*, S432–S433. doi: 10.1016/j.eurpsy.2017.01.418.

Chubak, J., Hawkes, R., Dudzik, C., Foose-Foster, J. M., Eaton, L., Johnson, R. H., & Macpherson, C. F. (2017). Pilot study of therapy dog visits for inpatient youth with cancer. *Journal of Pediatric Oncology Nursing, 34*(5), 331–341. doi: 10.1177/1043454217712983.

Connell, C. G., Tepper, D. L., Landry, O., & Bennett, P. C. (2019). Dogs in schools: The impact of specific human-dog interactions on reading ability in children aged 6–8 years. *Anthrozoos, 32*, 347–360.

Contalbrigo, L., De Santis, M., Toson, M., Montanaro, M., Farina, L., Costa, A., & Felice, A. N. (2017). The efficacy of dog assisted therapy in detained drug users: A pilot study in an Italian attenuated custody institute. *International Journal of Environmental Research and Public Health, 14*(7), 683–698. doi: 10.3390/ijerph14070683.

Cooley, L. F., & Barker, S. B. (2018). Canine-assisted therapy as an adjunct tool in the care of the surgical patient: A literature review and opportunity for research. *Alternative Therapies in Health and Medicine, 24*(3), 48.

Crossman, M. K. (2017). Effects of interactions with animals on human psychological distress. *Journal of Clinical Psychology, 73*, 761–784. doi: 10.1002/jclp.22410.

Crossman, M. K., Kazdin, A. E., & Knudson, K. (2015). Brief unstructured interaction with a dog reduces distress. *Anthrozoos, 28*(4), 649–659. doi: 10.1080/08927936.2015.1070008.

Crossman, M. K., Kazdin, A. E., Matijczak, A., Kitt, E. R., & Santos, L. R. (2018). The influence of interactions with dogs on affect, anxiety, and arousal in children. *Journal of Clinical Child & Adolescent Psychology*, Early online publication. doi: 10.1080/15374416.2018.1520119.

Delgado, C., Toukonen, M., & Wheeler, C. (2018). Effect of canine play interventions as a stress reduction strategy in college students. *Nurse Educator, 43*(3), 149–153. doi: 10.1097/NNE. 0000000000000451.

Dietz, T. J., Davis, D., & Pennings, J. (2012). Evaluating animal-assisted therapy in group treatment for child sexual abuse. *Journal of Child Sexual Abuse, 21*, 665–683. doi: 10.1080/10538712.2012.726700.

Elmaci, D. T., & Cevizci, S. (2015). Dog-assisted therapies and activities in rehabilitation of children with Cerebral Palsy and physical and mental disabilities. *International Journal of Environment Research and Public Health, 12*, 5046–5060. doi: 10I3390/ijerph120505046.

Grajfoner, D., Harte, E., Potter, L. M., & McGuigan, N. (2017). The effect of dog-assisted intervention on student well-being, mood, and anxiety. *International Journal of Environmental Research and Public Health, 14*(5), 483–494. doi: 10.3390/ijerph14050483.

Harper, C. M., Dong, Y., Thornhill, T. S., Wright, J., & Ready, J. (2015). Can therapy dogs improve pain and satisfaction after total joint arthroplasty? A randomized controlled trial. *Clinical Orthopaedics and Related Research, 473*(1), 372–379.

Hartwig, E. K. (2017). Building solutions in youth: Evaluation of the human-animal resilience therapy intervention. *Journal of Creativity in Mental Health, 12*(4), 468–481. doi: 10.1080/15401383.2017.1283281.

Herzog, H. (2011). The impact of pets on human health and psychological well-being: Fact, fiction, or hypothesis? *Current Directions in Psychological Science, 20*, 236–239. doi: 10.1 177/0963721411415220.

Herzog, H. (2014). Does animal-assisted therapy really work?: What clinical trials reveal about the effectiveness of four-legged therapists [online]. *Psychology Today*. Retrieved November 26, 2016, from www.psychologytoday.com/blog/animals-and-us/201411/does-animal-assisted-therapy-really-work

Hughes, K. (2002). See spot read. *Public Libraries, 41*(6), 328–330.

Kelly, M. A., & Cozzolino, C. A. (2015). Helping at-risk youth overcome trauma and substance abuse through animal-assisted therapy. *Contemporary Justice Review, 18*(4), 421–434. doi: 10.1080/10282580.2015.1093686.

Kirnan, J. P., Siminerio, S., & Wong, Z. (2016). The impact of a therapy dog reading program on children's reading skills and attitudes toward reading. *Early Childhood Education Journal, 44*(6), 637–651. doi: 10.1007/s10643-015-0747-9.

Kirnan, J., Ventresco, N. E., & Gardner, T. (2017). The impact of a therapy dog program on children's reading: Follow-up and extension to ELL students. *Early Childhood Education Journal, 46*(1), 103–116. doi: 10.1007/s10643-017-0844-z.

Kline, J. A., Fisher, M. A., Pettit, K. L., Linville, C. T., & Beck, A. M. (2019). Controlled clinical trial of canine therapy versus usual care to reduce patient anxiety in the emergency department. *PLoS One, 14*(01), 1–13. doi: 10.1371/journal.pone.0209232.

Lange, A., Cox, J., Bernert, D., & Jenkins, C. (2006/2007). Is counseling going to the dogs? An exploratory study related to the inclusion of an animal in group counseling with adolescents. *Journal of Creativity in Mental Health, 2*, 17–31. doi: 10.1300/J456v02n02_03.

Le Roux, M. C., Swartz, L., & Swart, E. (2014). The effect of an animal-assisted reading program on the reading rate, accuracy and comprehension of grade 3 students: A randomized control study. *Child & Youth Care Forum, 43*, 655–673. doi: 10.1007/s10566-014-9262-1.

Linder, D. E., Mueller, M. K., Gibbs, D. M., Alper, J. A., & Freeman, L. M. (2018). Effects of an animal-assisted intervention on reading skills and attitudes in second grade students. *Early Childhood Education Journal, 46*(3), 323–329. doi: 10.1007/s10643-017-0862-x.

Lutwack-Bloom, P., Wijewickrama, R., & Smith, B. (2005). Effects of pets versus people visits with nursing home residents. *Journal of Gerontological Social Work, 44*(3–4), 137–159. doi: 10.1300/J083v44n03_09.

Machová, K., Kejdanová, P., Bajtlerová, I., Procházková, R., Svobodová, I., & Mezian, K. (2018). Canine-assisted speech therapy for children with communication impairments: A randomized controlled trial. *Anthrozoös, 31*(5), 587–598. doi: 10.1080/08927936.2018.1505339.

Marino, L. (2012). Construct validity of animal-assisted therapy and activities: How important is the animal in AAT? *Anthrozoos, 25*, s139–s151. doi: 10.1016/S0887-6158(02)00199-8.

Nammalwar, R. B., & Rangeeth, P. (2018). A bite out of anxiety: Evaluation of animal-assisted activity on anxiety in children attending a pediatric dental outpatient unit. *Journal of the Indian Society of Pedodontics and Preventive Dentistry, 36,* 181–184.

Newlin, R. B. (2003). Paws for reading: An innovative program uses dogs to help kids read better. *School Library Journal, 49*(6), 43. doi: 10.1023/B:ECEJ.0000039638.607 14.5f.

Norton, M. J., Funaro, M. C., & Rojiani, R. (2018). Improving healthcare professionals' well-being through the use of therapy dogs. *Journal of Hospital Librarianship, 18*(3), 203–209. doi: 10.1080/15323269.2018.1471898.

Prothmann, A., Albrecht, K., Dietrich, S., Hornfeck, U., Stieber, S., & Ettrich, C. (2005). Analysis of child – dog play behavior in child psychiatry. *Anthrozoös, 18*(1), 43–58. doi: 10.2752/089279305785594261.

Prothmann, A., Bienert, M., & Ettrich, C. (2006). Dogs in child psychotherapy: Effects on state of mind. *Anthrozoös, 19*(3), 265–277.

Schwartz, A., & Patronek, G. (2002). Methodological issues in studying the anxiety-reducing effects of animals: Reflections from a pediatric dental study. *Anthrozoos, 15,* 290–299. doi: 10.2752/089279302786992432.

Shubert, J. (2012, April–June). Therapy dogs and stress management assistance during disasters. *U.S. Army Medical Department Journal,* 74–78.

Thodberg, K., Sørensen, L. U., Videbech, P. B., Poulsen, P. H., Houbak, B., Damgaard, V. . . . Christensen, J. W. (2016). Behavioral responses of nursing home residents to visits from a person with a dog, a robot seal or a toy cat. *Anthrozoös, 29,* 107–121. doi: 10.1080/08927936.2015.108901.

Ward-Griffin, E., Klaiber, P., Collins, H. K., Owens, R. L., Coren, S., & Chen, F. S. (2018). Petting away pre-exam stress: The effect of therapy dog sessions on student well-being. *Stress and Health, 34*(3), 468–473. doi: 10.1002/smi.2804.

Wesley, M. C., Minatrea, N. B., & Watson, J. C. (2009). Animal-assisted therapy in the treatment of substance dependence. *Anthrozoös, 22*(2), 137–148. doi: 10.2752/1753 03709X434167.

Wilson, E. O. (1984). *Biophilia.* Cambridge, MA: Harvard University Press.

2   What Are Canine-Assisted Interventions?

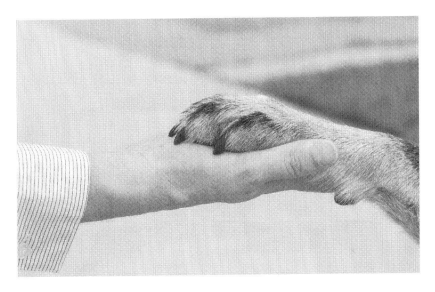

Figure 2.1 Human-animal interaction.

The aim of this chapter is to provide readers with a foundational understanding of the human-animal bond, theoretical explanations for human-animal interactions (HAIs), the benefits of canine-assisted interventions (CAIs), and types of CAIs. This chapter explores the goals and motives for why we do what we do in the practice of CAIs. Consider the following scenario.

Scenario

Phyllis has had a busy week. Within the span of 1 week, she has had the opportunity to interact with several different therapy dogs. On Sunday, Phyllis visited her mother, who is cared for at a memory care facility. During this visit, a volunteer CAI team trained to work on wellness goals stopped by her mom's room. Phyllis's mom asked if the therapy dog could sit with her on the bed so that her mom could pet the dog. The handler saw that there were no safety issues, such as cords or medication near the bed, and allowed the therapy dog to sit on the bed for a few minutes. Phyllis enjoyed seeing her mom pet the therapy dog and talk about how much she enjoyed having pets over the years. On Monday, Phyllis went to work as a schoolteacher. Every Monday, a CAI team trained to work on academic goals visits the campus to work with students who are struggling with math. After only three months, one of Phyllis's students who has been completing math assignments in the presence of a therapy dog has increased his math skills, as evidenced by a higher score on a recent math exam. Her student is excited to tell his mom that he is getting better grades in math and tells Phyllis that he loves completing math assignments with Pickles, the math tutoring dog. On Wednesday, Phyllis went with her husband to the physical therapy clinic, where he is working on rehabilitating his arm after a serious fall. The physical therapist works with a therapy dog who has been trained to work on rehabilitation goals. The physical therapist has the dog sit in different places to help Phyllis's husband extend his reach as he pets and interacts with the dog. Back at school on Friday, the school counselor arrived at Phyllis's classroom with a therapy dog who is trained to work with the school counselor on mental health goals. The school counselor asked to see one of Phyllis's students, who is coping with grief after the death of her father six months earlier. As Phyllis watches her student, the therapy dog, and the school counselor walk down the hallway to the counselor's office, Phyllis reflects on how grateful she is for the ways in which therapy dogs have supported the people she cares about this week.

Questions for Reflection and Discussion

1. What benefits do the therapy dogs bring in each of these settings?
2. Do all therapy dog teams provide the same services?

Foundations of HAIs

Throughout history, humans and animals have lived among one another. Early evidence of HAIs revealed that humans utilized animals for fundamental aspects of human life (DeLoache, Pickard, & LoBue, 2011). Animal bodies were used for food, tools, jewelry, clothes, and materials. Animals also served in other roles, such as transportation, load carriers, and herders (Mullin, 2002). All of these animal roles allowed humans to not only survive but to thrive in their communities. Over time, perceptions of HAIs have evolved. Animals now interact with humans in more intimate systems. HAIs are the ways in which humans and animals behave and associate in the presence of one another.

Human-Animal Bond

The human-animal bond is defined as a

mutually beneficial and dynamic relationship between people and animals that is influenced by behaviors considered essential to the health and well-being of both. The bond includes, but is not limited to emotional, psychological, and physical interactions of people, animals, and the environment.

(American Veterinary Medical Association, 2018, para. 2)

One way to view the human-animal bond is through the lens of pet ownership. According to an online survey of more than 20 countries by Growth for Knowledge (2018), 33% of people are dog owners. The American Pet Products Association (APPA, 2018) reported that 68% of U.S. households own a pet, with almost half of U.S. households having a dog as a pet (48%). APPA also reported the following findings:

- 81% of pet owners believe that having a pet promotes good health.
- 85% believe that pet affection is beneficial.
- 71% believe that pets bring their family closer together.
- 33% believe their pet helps them increase their exercise.
- 80% believe their pet increases their mood.
- 66% believe their pet decreases stress.

These figures show that a majority of pet owners view having a pet as beneficial to health, mood, stress level, and family bonding. Pets provide humans with multiple opportunities to connect with animals, the environment, and other people. Research by Bao and Schreer (2016) indicated that pet owners reported greater life satisfaction than non-pet owners. There is ample support affirming that pet owners perceive several benefits to having a pet in their home.

Theoretical Explanations for HAIs

Researchers have proposed numerous theories to explain why humans seek interactions with animals, how humans associate with animals, and how human-animal relations yield positive effects on human well-being (Beetz, 2017; Kruger & Serpell, 2010). Prevalent theories in CAI literature include biophilia, neurobiology, and social support. In this section we'll explore these theoretical perspectives undergirding HAI.

As mentioned in Chapter 1, Wilson (1984) promoted the concept of biophilia as the "the urge to affiliate with other forms of life" (p. 85). The biophilia theory suggests that human strive to connect with nature—mountains and valleys, celestial spaces, and even animals. Researchers proposed that the resting behavior of animals promotes feelings of security in humans and is known as the "biophilia effect" (Julius, Beetz, Kotrschal, Turner, & Uvnäs-Moberg, 2013). The biophilia effect may explain the mechanisms by which interactions with animals decrease stress and anxiety (Barker & Dawson, 1998). Some studies have supported the biophilia theory by submitting that animals are effective in attracting and holding human attention (Barker & Dawson, 1998). In order to maintain connectedness in social environments, humans have an implicit need to make sense of the actions of animals (Epley, Waytz, & Cacioppo, 2007). Anthropomorphism is a process in which people attribute humanlike characteristics to animals (e.g., animals greet humans, animals want to be hugged). In a study on self-disclosure with dogs by Evans-Wilday, Hall, Hogue, and Mills (2018), researchers indicated that dog owners were more likely to talk to their dogs than a confidant about depression, jealousy, anxiety, calmness, apathy, and fear-based emotions. Furthermore, dog owners were more willing to talk about jealousy and apathy with their dog than with their partner or a confidant (Evans-Wilday et al., 2018). This anthropomorphic affinity toward human characteristics in dogs and interacting in humanlike ways with dogs may explain and increase the appeal of CAIs.

A neurobiological explanation for HAIs is the activation of the oxytocin system. Researchers suggest that the neuroendocrine systems that produce hormones, such as oxytocin, offer insight into reciprocal processes that can increase social interactions, buffer stress responses, and enhance the effects of social support (Carter & Porges, 2016; Heinrichs, Baumgartner, Kirschbaum, & Ehlert, 2003). In 2000, Odendaal sought to gain medical support for HAIs by investigating six neurochemicals associated with affiliation and decreased blood pressure in humans and dogs before and after a positive interaction. Results indicated that neurochemicals such as oxytocin and dopamine increased significantly in both humans and dogs. This outcome suggests that both humans and dogs experience connection and attention-seeking behaviors through HAIs. Results also indicated that positive interaction with a dog can produce a significant decrease in blood pressure between 5 and 24 minutes after an interaction. This finding proposes that HAIs with dogs can have positive effects after a relatively short interaction, and thus the need for long interactions (e.g., 60 minutes) is not required to experience positive effects. Beetz (2017) emphasized that the activation of oxytocin through HAIs can not only produce positive effects, such as lower stress, but also may explain outcomes in studies that measure the benefits of HAI (e.g., reductions in heart rate).

Another theory that supports the phenomenon of HAI is social support. Animals can be catalysts for HAI and may accelerate the relationship-building process between clients and handlers (Kruger & Serpell, 2010). Often described as "man's best friend," dogs have the ability to be facilitators of social interactions and function as sources of social support for humans (Grandgeorge & Hausberger, 2011). Wood (2011) promoted the idea that animals increase social capital for humans. Drawing on her own research, Wood proposed that companion animals foster social capital through seven modalities: (1) facilitating interactions and relationships with others, (2) showing empathy and how humans relate to others, (3) promoting civic engagement and community involvement, (4) fostering tolerance and trust, (5) forming social networks of support, (6) getting "out and about" in the community, and (7) "doing the right thing" for the community. In addition to increasing social capital, Zilcha-Mano, Mikulincer, and Shaver (2011) proposed that animals involved in HAIs can influence and respond to clients' unmet attachment needs, individual differences in insecure attachment, coping skills, and responsiveness to therapy. For people who don't have dogs or access to dogs, CAIs can fill the void of social support. For example, college students missing their dogs at home or feeling homesick from their families can connect with therapy dogs and their handlers on campus to fill their need for social interaction. Similarly, elder care recipients, such as residents at an assisted living facility, may not receive regular visits from family members or friends and appreciate visits by CAI teams who provide an opportunity for interaction. These perspectives and related examples affirm the role that dogs can play in increasing social capital for their human companions and facilitate social interactions as part of HAIs.

Benefits of CAIs

The internet is buzzing with videos, stories, and pictures of how therapy dogs make a difference in people's lives. Anecdotal stories and positive experiences with dogs influence our belief that dogs have a positive impact on people; however, it's important that structured interactions with dogs are guided by best practice principles and grounded in strong science. Researchers have worked hard to establish and identify scientific findings attesting to the benefits of HAIs, and CAIs specifically. Next, we'll review the physical, emotional, social, educational, and contextual benefits of CAIs.

Physical Benefits

Numerous studies have investigated the physical benefits of CAIs. Researchers have explored the impact of CAIs in alleviating stress in medical and forensic settings with children. In a study on the presence of a dog during a physical examination with young children, Nagengast, Baun, Megel, and Michael Leibowitz (1997) found statistically significant reductions in systolic and mean arterial pressure, heart rate, and behavioral distress, suggesting that therapy dogs reduce indicators of stress. Similarly, research by Tsai, Friedmann, and Thomas (2010) indicated decreased systolic blood pressure in hospitalized children after interaction with a therapy dog, with continuation of decreased blood pressure a few minutes after the CAI. Braun, Stangler, Narveson, and Pettingell (2009) asserted that the presence of a therapy dog in a pediatric setting was an effective modality for reducing pain in children. Outcomes from their study indicated that children who interacted with a therapy dog reported pain reduction that was four times greater than the comparison group of children who relaxed quietly for 15 minutes without a therapy dog present. In a study on children undergoing forensic interviews for alleged sexual abuse, Krause-Parello and Friedmann (2014) found that salivary biomarkers for stress were lower when a dog was present with children. Outcomes from their study also revealed that even with older children during longer forensic interviews, heart rate decreased and children experienced a greater reduction in their heart rate when a therapy dog was present. Combined, these studies suggest that the involvement of a dog in medical settings with children can foster positive physical benefits.

Researchers have also identified physical benefits for adults. In a study on early ambulation (i.e., walking) for chronic heart failure patients, Abate, Zucconi, and Boxer (2011) reported increased motivation to walk and increased walking distance. Similar to Braun, Stangler, Narveson, and Pettingell's (2009) findings reported previously, chronic pain patients reported significant reductions in pain and emotional distress after interacting with a therapy dog (Marcus, et al., 2012). Findings from these studies suggest that interacting with therapy dogs is not uniquely beneficial for children and can yield positive physical benefits for adults as well.

Emotional Benefits

Therapy dogs can also positively impact people's emotions. Barker and Dawson (1998) reported a significant reduction in anxiety scores for patients with psychiatric disorders after interacting with a dog. In a meta-analysis investigating the effectiveness of animal-assisted interactions (AAIs) in reducing depression, outcomes revealed that AAIs are effective in significantly reducing depression with medium effect sizes (Souter & Miller, 2007). CAIs have also been shown to decrease depression and anxiety in seniors in assisted living

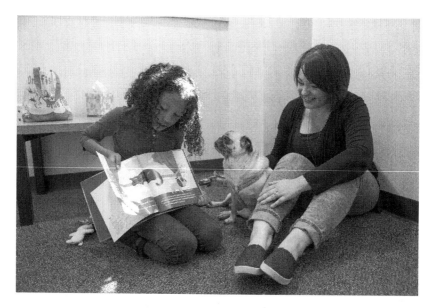

Figure 2.2 Therapy dog Stella provides emotional support to children in schools with her school counselor partner, Missy Whitsett.

facilities (Colombo, Buono, Smania, Raviola, & De Leo, 2006) and increase self-esteem and self-determination of Taiwanese inpatients with schizophrenia (Chu, Liu, Sun, & Lin, 2009). Campbell, Smith, Tumilty, Cameron, and Treharne (2016) explored how dog walking influences perspectives of health and well-being in healthy adults. Findings from this study indicated that the emotional connection between humans and dogs increased inherent motivation to exercise (i.e., dog walking) and enhanced psychological well-being.

Social Benefits

When one considers the theory that dogs increase social support and social capital, it's comes as no surprise that researchers have studied the social benefits of CAIs. In a literature review of AAI with psychiatric patients, Rossetti and King (2010) noted that AAIs can significantly improve socialization in psychiatric patients, as well as provide a variety of psychological benefits. For patients with schizophrenia, Barak, Savorai, Mavashev, and Beni (2001) identified that interaction with a therapy dog increased socialization, daily living activities, and quality of life. CAIs can also provide support for loneliness. Residents in long-term care facilities participated in a study in which they received 6 weeks of CAI, with 30-minute sessions in either individual or group settings (Banks & Banks, 2005). Residents receiving individual canine-assisted activity (CAA) sessions had lower loneliness scores when compared to residents receiving CAA in a group setting. These outcomes indicate that individual CAA sessions may be more effective for this population.

Research on the social outcomes of CAIs with children have produced promising results. Findings from Schuck, Emmerson, Fine, and Lakes (2015) revealed that children diagnosed with attention deficit hyperactivity disorder (ADHD) who were involved in a cognitive-behavioral therapy (CBT) group with a therapy dog demonstrated lower severity of ADHD symptoms than children in the CBT group without a therapy dog. In a study of children with developmental disorders, Martin and Farnum (2002) discovered that children were more playful and aware of their social environment when a therapy dog was present. Thus, there are a number of social benefits arising from interacting with therapy dogs.

Educational Benefits

Fine and Gee (2017) argue that dogs in classrooms provide a host of benefits, such as increased empathy and responsibility, decreased anxiety and stress in the classroom, enhanced literacy skills, and improved classroom behavior. In their research on the effects of animals in educational settings on children's academic skills, Gee and colleagues (e.g., Gee, Church, & Altobelli, 2010; Gee, Crist, & Carr, 2010; Gee, Gould, Swanson, & Wagner, 2012) found that, in the presence of a real dog, young children follow instructions attentively, make less errors when performing a cognitive task, and focus and perform motor skills faster with animate objects, such as animals and people, than inanimate objects, such as things or places. One explanation for these findings is that animals motivate students for learning (Rud & Beck, 2003).

Researchers have also found that dogs improve psychosocial skills. In a qualitative study of children with emotional disorders, researchers found that the presence of a dog in the classroom increased students' emotional stability and attitudes toward school and facilitated student learning of responsibility, respect, and empathy (Anderson & Olson, 2006). Hergovich, Monshi, Semmler, and Zieglmayer (2002) found that students exhibited higher social integration and less aggression when a dog was present in the classroom. In a study on teachers' experiences with humane education, Daly and Suggs (2010) found that teachers reported that having pets in the classroom contributed to increases in children's empathy and socioemotional development. Combined, these studies suggest that the presence of a dog in a classroom can produce both academic and psychosocial benefits for students.

Benefits in College Settings

Transitioning from high school to a college setting can be especially challenging for young adults. Therapy dogs within this context are thought "to temporarily fill the absence of previous support systems and be a catalyst for establishing new relationships" (Adamle, Riley, & Carlson, 2009, p. 545). A number of studies have explored the impact of therapy dog programs on college student well-being, including the reduction of homesickness (Binfet & Passmore, 2016) and stress (e.g., Barker, Barker, McCain, & Schubert, 2016; Crossman, Kazdin, & Knudson, 2015, Ward-Griffin et al., 2018). In a study assessing the effects of an 8-week CAI with first-year college students, Binfet and Passmore (2016) identified a reduction in participant-reported homesickness and increases in life satisfaction and connectedness to campus. In a follow-up study, Binfet (2017) investigated the effects of a single-session, group-administered CAI on student well-being. Findings from this study indicated significant reductions in perceived stress and homesickness and significant improvements in sense of school belonging. Together, these studies suggest that both short-term and more sustained interaction with a therapy dog can improve student well-being within the context of a college campus.

Several studies have explored the influence of CAIs on students who are preparing for final exams. An experimental trial by Pendry, Carr, Roeter, and Vandagriff (2018) proposed that 10 minutes of CAI increased levels of contentment and decreased levels of anxiety and irritability in college students preparing for final examinations. In another study, college students who interacted with a therapy dog reported significantly lower stress scores, with large effect sizes, when compared to a control group (Barker et al., 2016). Banks, McCoy, and Trzcinski (2018) also explored the influence of CAIs on college students during an exam period. Findings from this study noted that interacting with therapy dogs reduced state anxiety and perceived stress but did not

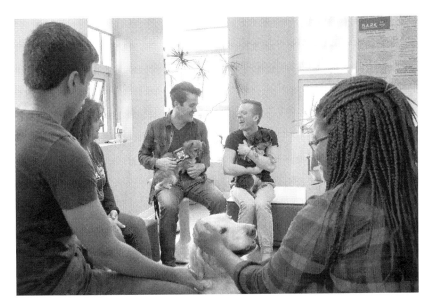

Figure 2.3 Canine-assisted activity: college students connecting with dogs.

positively affect cognitive outcomes, such as sustained attention and mind wandering. Overall, these studies on supporting the well-being of college students during final exams suggest that CAIs reduce anxiety and stress.

Benefits in Mental Health Settings

Levinson (1969) was a pioneer in the CAI field through his writings about incorporating his dog, Jingles, into therapy sessions. Levinson discovered that Jingles appeared to create a more relaxed environment for children, which encouraged self-disclosure. The current literature base for CAIs has advanced Levinson's initial anecdotal research by demonstrating a myriad of positive indicators for clients. Prothmann, Bienert, and Ettrich (2006) explored the influence of CAIs on the state of mind in children receiving inpatient psychiatric treatment. The findings revealed that children in the CAI treatment group had significantly higher scores in all four state of mind subscales: vitality, intraemotional balance, social extroversion, and alertness. Prothmann and colleagues (2006) emphasized that "incorporating a dog could catalyze psychotherapeutic work with children and adolescents" (p. 1).

To empirically assess the effects of having therapy dogs participate in individual counseling, Hartwig (2017) facilitated a randomized comparison trial in which adolescents participated in 10 weeks of individual counseling using the Human-Animal Resilience Therapy (HART; Hartwig, 2017) curriculum. The HART curriculum, composed of a series of interactive activities, was used to help participants work toward their counseling goals. The findings revealed statistically significant differences between pretest and posttest scores for anxiety, depression, and disruptive behavior inventories for participants working with and without therapy dogs. Further support for the integration of therapy dogs in counseling is found in a study by Lange, Cox, Bernert, and Jenkins (2006/2007). The inclusion of a dog in an anger management group for adolescents resulted in a host of positive outcomes for participants: a calming effect, humor relief, an increased feeling of safety, empathy, and a higher motivation to attend sessions (Lange et al., 2006/2007). Research by Hanselman (2001) found adolescents who worked with a therapy dog in an anger management group demonstrated reduced apprehension. Together, the findings from these studies indicate the positive influence of dogs in counseling adolescents.

Researchers have also examined the role of CAIs in inpatient settings. In a study by Stefanini, Martino, Allori, Galeotti, and Tani (2015), adolescents with acute mental disorders who interacted with a dog reported significant improvement in global functioning and increased school attendance when compared to a no-dog control group. In a recent study of adolescents in residential care who were challenged by traumatic childhood experiences and mental health issues, adolescents who participated in 12 weeks of counseling with a therapy dog demonstrated higher levels of secure attachment when compared to participants in a control group (Balluerka, Muela, Amiano, & Caldentey, 2014). Mental health-based CAIs in both outpatient and inpatient settings have contributed to clinical progress with adolescent clients.

Mental health practitioners themselves see potential benefits to working with animals in clinical settings. Lutsky-Cohen and Schneider (2017) indicated that practitioners perceived the following benefits of AAIs: clients experience comfort, a positive effect on client health; clients are more relaxed with an animal present; animals can be entertainment; animals can provide a distraction from painful topics; it's easier for clients to open up; clients are more motivated to return to therapy; and it's easier for practitioners to build a relationship with a client when an animal is present. In this same study, practitioners shared perceived benefits of AAI for therapists. These included the following: animals can have a positive impact on therapists' health, the work atmosphere is more relaxing and entertaining, animals improve the therapeutic process, therapists are able to take their pets to work, and therapists may feel less lonely at work. CAIs appear to have potential benefits for both clients and practitioners.

Contraindications of AAIs

Although there are numerous and varied reported benefits of AAIs in the anthrozoological literature, there is also evidence that AAIs do not result in desired outcomes and that much more research is needed. In a meta-analysis of studies on the effects of animal-assisted therapy (AAT), Nimer and Lundahl

(2007) identified AAT as an adjunct to other interventions, rather than a standalone provision, and suggested that AAT produced moderate outcomes. Nimer and Lundahl advised that considerable variance exists in AAT research and that more research is needed to more accurately identify the impact of AAT interventions. Souter and Miller (2007) echoed the need for more rigorous research in the field of AAI by recommending higher standards for research designs, such as random assignment, the use of physiological measures (e.g., heart rate, blood pressure), and the need to research the long-term effects of AAIs.

There have been additional and more recent calls for methodologically stronger AAI research. Herzog (2011) suggested that a universal "pet effect" of the positive impact of pets on human health is more of a hypothesis than a substantiated fact (p. 236). Herzog (2011, p. 236) argues,

> Most pet owners believe that their companion animals are good for them. Personal convictions, however, do not constitute scientific evidence. Claims about the medical and psychological benefits of living with animals need to be subjected to the same standards of evidence as a new drug, medical device, or form of psychotherapy.

In a systematic review of AAIs, Marino (2012) found only moderate and broad effects. Marino argues that research is needed that provides definitive conclusions regarding whether the involvement of a live animal is necessary for positive therapeutic effects. Serpell, McCune, Gee, and Griffin (2017, p. 223) noted that

> practical challenges to AAI research include issues of study design and methodology, the heterogeneity of both AAI recipients and the animals participating in these interventions, the welfare of these animals, and the unusual pressure from the public and media to report and publish positive findings.

As the field of CAI advances, these researchers argue for stronger research designs and methodology. We contend that CAI-themed research can profit from clearly identified standards for CAI training and assessment and explore this topic in more depth in Chapter 10. Our goal in writing this book is to identify best practices for CAIs that will increase the consistency of the screening, training, and assessment of CAI teams across all contexts—whether they participate in volunteer or professional settings or in research exploring the effects of CAIs on human well-being.

Types of HAIs With Canines

The term "animal-assisted therapy" has become overused and muddled. News reports, online videos, and even volunteer organizations refer to a variety of services involving human-animal teams as "animal-assisted therapy," even when the human volunteers are not licensed therapists and are not providing goal-oriented therapeutic services. An example of this confusion was found in Chapter 1, where the public's perception of the lines differentiating therapy dogs from service dogs can become blurred. As the field of CAI expands and develops, a clear understanding of the different types of human-canine interactions is needed.

AAI is an umbrella term for the myriad of services provided by human-animal teams. The International Association for Human-Animal Interaction Organizations (IAHAIO, 2018) defines an AAI as a "goal oriented and structured intervention that intentionally includes or incorporates animals in health, education and human service (e.g., social work) for the purpose of therapeutic gains in humans" (p. 5). This definition clearly articulates that AAIs are structured (i.e., planned) and are focused on a goal to improve human wellness. This definition also recognizes that the animal is *involved* in the intervention. The level of animal involvement could be the mere presence of an animal, such as a facility dog at a funeral home, or the animal being asked to move or interact with a client, such as a horse who provides therapeutic riding to children with unique abilities. In Figure 2.4, we attempt to clarify the various roles therapy dogs play in CAIs through our CAI Pathways to Well-Being model.

Canine-Assisted Activities (CAAs)

In our opening scenario at the beginning of this chapter, the CAI team visiting Phyllis's mother at the memory care facility was an example of a canine-assisted activity (CAA). CAAs are the most common form of CAIs. CAAs are informal human-canine interactions that are focused on broad wellness goals, such as comfort, social interaction, and stress reduction. CAAs are typically services provided by volunteer CAI teams. This means that the handler

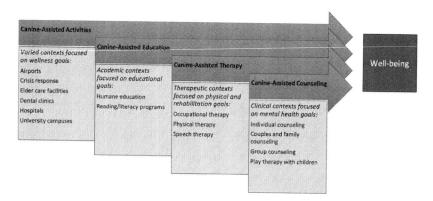

Figure 2.4 Pathways to well-being model.

Box 2.1   CAA Overview

CAA *handlers*: Volunteers
CAA *time frame*: Brief (10 to 15 minutes)
CAA *service examples*:

- teams who visit residents in memory care facilities
- teams who visit children receiving chemotherapy in hospitals
- teams with canines whom students can pet and interact with during finals week at universities
- teams who visit displaced residents in shelters after a hurricane or who support victims and mourners after a public tragedy

---

does not need to be a specialist in a certain field. Although CAA teams are often referred to as "therapy dog teams," they generally do not provide actual mental health therapy, but rather provide comfort and support to people in need. Box 2.1 provides an overview and examples of CAA services.

When compared to other CAIs, several positive features of CAAs emerge. CAAs generally require less training for both the human and dog. Thus, people who are interested in volunteering with their dogs and have dogs that would be a good fit for CAAs can go through the process to become volunteer teams in a relatively short time frame and without intensive training that other CAI practitioners may need for the clients they serve. Further, CAA services are mobile. CAA teams visit a variety of settings—airports, universities, summer camps, and hospices—whereas canine-assisted therapy (CAT) and canine-assisted counseling (CAC) services are less mobile and tend to focus their services in specific places, such as clinics or private practice offices.

CAA Illustration

One example of a CAA is found in airports. Many airports across North America have introduced therapy dog programs to alleviate stress in travelers. Some of these CAA programs are found at Los Angeles International Airport's Pups Unstressing Passengers (PUP), Vancouver International Airport's The Less Airport Stress Initiative (LASI), Sacramento International Airport's Boarding Area Relaxation Corp (BARC), Denver International Airport's Canine Airport Therapy Squad (CATS), San Francisco International Airport's Wag Brigade, and Miami International Airport's Miami Hound Machine (Associated Press, 2018; Fodors, 2018). In these programs, CAA teams circulate in waiting areas and in different concourses, available for travelers to interact with the teams. Many teams carry trading cards that provide information about the therapy dog's favorite treat or pet peeve.

Fodors (2018) reported that airport CAA teams have supported passengers who have a fear of flying, are traveling to or from a funeral, or are missing their beloved pets at home. In Chapter 8 we will explore training and assessment considerations for teams working in unique contexts, such as airports, as work within different contexts requires nuanced skills on the part of both the handler and the therapy dog.

Canine-Assisted Education (CAE)

In our scenario at the beginning of the chapter, the CAI team working on math skills with Phyllis's student was an example of canine-assisted education (CAE). The American Veterinary Medical Association (2018, para. 6) defines animal-assisted education as a "planned and structured intervention directed and/or delivered by educational and related service professional with specific academic or educational goals." CAE often occurs in a school or classroom setting in which the CAI team can support students working toward academic goals. CAE can be provided to groups, such as an entire third-grade class, or to individuals, such as a college student working on public speaking skills. The instructor can serve as the dog's handler or the instructor can invite a CAI team to participate in classroom activities. One type of educational goal in which CAE is especially valuable is humane education—teaching children about animal welfare and how to treat animals. There are a variety of ways in which dogs can support academic goals. Box 2.2 provides an overview and examples of CAE services.

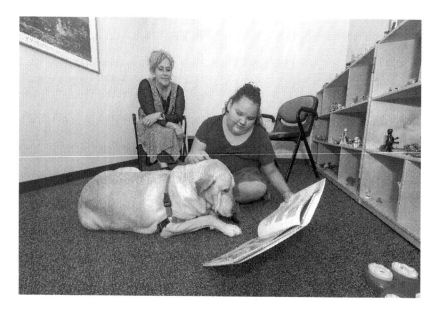

Figure 2.5 Canine-assisted education: child reading to a therapy dog.

Box 2.2   CAE Overview

CAE handlers: Teachers, professors, and volunteers
CAE time frame: 15–60 minutes, depending on the length of the educational activity
CAE service examples:

- reading programs
- humane education
- classroom guidance lessons

CAE Illustration

One of the most common CAE services is seen in canine-assisted literacy programs. One goal in canine literacy programs is to increase a child's reading fluency by allowing the child to read to a dog—a nonjudgmental being who will not correct the child. Another goal of canine literacy is to lower the stress that children sometimes feel when reading aloud. Let's imagine that 8-year-old James is struggling with his reading skills and self-confidence and is reading well below his grade level. James's teacher has coordinated for James to work with a volunteer CAI team, Mrs. Norris and Sully, a Labrador. James and the CAI team meet in the library for 30 minutes every week. Mrs. Norris has James choose several books at his current reading level and James reads the books to Sully. Sully may choose to look at James, look around the library, or sleep while James is reading to him. After 8 weeks of reading to Sully, James's reading level is reassessed, and the results reveal that James has increased both his reading competency and the confidence with which he now reads aloud. We'll explore this topic further in Chapter 8 when we examine the training and assessment implications of having a CAI team work within the context of an elementary school.

Canine-Assisted Therapy (CAT)

Another form of CAIs is canine-assisted therapy (CAT). In our scenario at the beginning of the chapter, the CAI team supporting Phyllis's husband's recovery at the physical therapy clinic was an example of CAT. CATs are interventions administered by professional rehabilitation therapists in therapeutic contexts that are focused on rehabilitation or physical goals. IAHAIO (2018) describes that AAT practitioners must be formally trained, have the necessary degree or licensure, and have proficiency within the scope of their professional practice. CAT service providers typically provide some form of therapy, such as occupational or physical therapy, or provide services within specific health settings, such as pediatric nurses or autism behavioral specialists.

Box 2.3   CAT Overview

CAT *practitioners*: Occupational therapists, physical therapists, nurses, and autism behavior specialists
CAT *time frame*: Brief (10 to 15 minutes) to full sessions (50 minutes to 1 hour)
CAT *service examples*:

- mobility training as part of physical therapy
- social interaction sessions for children with autism
- pain relief intervention for pediatric hospital patients

A major distinction between CAA and CAT services is that CAT occurs in a professional setting and is facilitated by a professional or a professional working in partnership with a volunteer CAI team. If a professional chooses to partner with a volunteer CAI team, then the team would be present while the professional (e.g., a physical therapist) is working with a client. This allows the professional to focus on the therapy intervention while the CAI team provides support to the client and promotes HAI during the intervention. CAT interventions may be brief, such as having a therapy dog present while a patient is receiving an immunization, or may be longer, such as a therapy dog being present for the entire hour-long occupational therapy session. Box 2.3 provides an overview and examples of CAT services.

CAT Illustration

An example of CAT is when a therapy dog is incorporated into occupational therapy to improve the quality of life of clients. Occupational therapists help clients work on and master daily living tasks, such as getting dressed, brushing teeth, and preparing food. Clients may need occupational therapy due to developmental delays, an injury, or a stroke. A client who has experienced a stroke can practice gross motor skills by petting and brushing a dog. The client can also practice fine motor skills by putting small dog treats into a puzzle toy for the dog. Having a therapy dog present and involved in therapy can be motivating for a client. Likewise, receiving petting, brushing, or treats can be a positive experience for the dog. This example of using CAT in occupational therapy demonstrates a positive and reciprocal HAI.

Canine-Assisted Counseling (CAC)

Canine-assisted counseling (CAC) is a form of CAI within the context of therapeutic services to treat clients' mental health. In our scenario at the beginning of the chapter, we saw an example of CAC in which a CAI team, composed of a school counselor and her therapy dog, worked with a student on mental health goals. There are a variety of terms that can be used to refer to canine-assisted mental health services. We use the term CAC in this book because this term can be used by a variety of mental health professionals, including counselors, psychologists, marriage and family therapists, and social workers. Hartwig (2019, para. 1) defines animal-assisted counseling as "a goal-directed process in which a trained mental health practitioner-animal team work together to help clients resolve mental health and behavioral challenges and achieve growth using the therapeutic powers of human-animal interaction." There are two ways in which CAC is distinguished from CAT: (1) CAC is focused on mental health goals, whereas CAT is focused on rehabilitation goals, and (2) CAC practitioners are mental health providers, such as licensed professional counselors, psychologists, marriage and family therapists, or clinical social workers, whereas CAT providers are physical, occupational, speech-language, or behavior intervention therapists.

CAC interventions typically take place over the course of a full 45-minute to 1-hour session. In order to facilitate CAC, practitioners must learn how to work with a therapy dog for an extended period of time, teach clients how to interact with the dog, create clinical treatment plans, and develop counseling interventions that include the dog and help the client work toward clinical goals. Due to the sustained involvement of the therapy dog and the specialized skills that CAC practitioners must learn, CAC involves more training

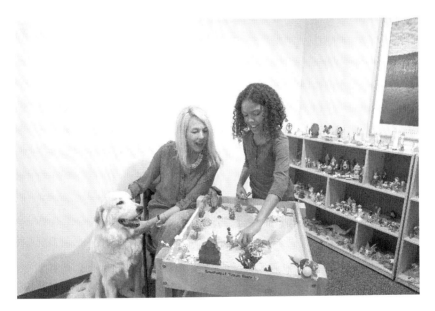

Figure 2.6 Canine-assisted counseling: Kristy Donaldson and therapy dog Willow facilitate sandtray play with a child.

Box 2.4   CAC Overview

CAC *practitioners*: Professional counselors, psychologists, marriage and family therapists, and clinical social workers
CAC *time frame*: Full session (45 minutes to 1 hour)
CAC *service examples*:

- individual counseling for trauma
- grief groups for teens who have experienced the death of a loved one
- play therapy for children

---

than CAA volunteers routinely receive. In light of this specialized training and the complexities of incorporating a therapy dog into the delivery of counseling services provided to clients, we have devoted Chapter 6 to an in-depth exploration of this topic. Box 2.4 provides an overview and examples of CAC services.

CAC Illustration

To illustrate a CAC intervention, let's imagine that a licensed professional counselor and his therapy dog, Willow, are working with a 12-year-old client who is grieving the death of her mother. In CAC, it's important to have a clinical goal for each client with interventions that involve the therapy dog—that is, there is a reason behind the clinician's decision to incorporate a therapy dog into the client's treatment plan and it is thought the incorporation of the dog into the session will facilitate the client attaining her or his goals. The goals for our young client here might be to develop three adaptive coping skills for grieving the loss of her mother. One CAC intervention that could help this client develop coping skills and involves Willow is called the "Challenge Tunnel." The Challenge Tunnel intervention uses a play tunnel and sticky notes as resources. The counselor would ask the client to brainstorm all the ways in which she feels challenged by the death of her mother (e.g., her mom isn't there to help her with homework, say good night). The client would then write each challenge on a sticky note and put the notes somewhere around the outside of the play tunnel. Then the counselor would ask the client to see if she can get Willow through the challenge tunnel—past all of the challenges that the client has experienced. The client would have to find ways to encourage Willow through the tunnel, such as the client crawling through the tunnel first or using treats to encourage Willow to go through the tunnel. Then the counselor and the client would process how Willow overcame the challenge of getting through the tunnel (e.g., Willow received help and encouragement from the client, Willow was willing to try and go through the tunnel). Together, they would discuss what skills the client could try over the next week that might be helpful coping skills for grief (e.g., getting support from others, listening to some of her mom's favorite music, and making a memory collage of pictures of her mom). In this example, Willow was an active part of a CAC intervention that helped the client work toward her clinical goal.

Conclusion

As you can see, there is an abundance of evidence-based outcomes attesting to the benefits of CAIs. That said, we also recognize the need for additional research and the refinement of standards to support the incorporation of CAIs to support well-being across varied contexts. Now that we have provided an overview of CAIs and their pathway to supporting well-being and established how CAIs can help clients physically, emotionally, socially, and contextually, it's important to look at what factors help create a strong CAI team. More specifically, what attributes, skills, and dispositions make a strong and effective CAI team?

References

Abate, S. V., Zucconi, M., & Boxer, B. A. (2011). Impact of canine-assisted ambulation on hospitalized chronic heart failure patients' ambulation outcomes and satisfaction: A pilot study. *Journal of Cardiovascular Nursing, 26,* 224–230.

Adamle, K., Riley, T., & Carlson, T. (2009). Evaluating college student interest in pet therapy. *Journal of American College Health, 57,* 545–548.

American Pet Products Association (APPA). (2018). 2017–2018 APPA National Pet Owners Survey statistics: Pet ownership and annual expenses. Retrieved October 31, 2018, from https://americanpetproducts.org/press_industrytrends.asp and https://vimeo.com/orangetreeps/review/214716969/38f274fe6d

American Veterinary Medical Association (AVMA). (2018). The human-animal interaction and human-animal bond. Retrieved December 17, 2018, from www.avma.org/KB/Policies/Pages/The-Human-Animal-Bond.aspx

Anderson, K. L., & Olson, M. R. (2006). The value of a dog in a classroom of children with severe emotional disorders. *Anthrozoös, 19*(1), 35–49. doi: 10.2752/0892793 06785593919.

Associated Press. (2018). *Therapy dogs to calm passengers at Miami airport. AP Regional State Report—Florida.* Associated Press DBA Press Association. Retrieved December 17, 2018, from www.apnews.com/d3a572da9fb04f67802346ea295cb084

Balluerka, N., Muela, A., Amiano, N., & Caldentey, M. A. (2014). Influence of animal-assisted therapy (AAT) on the attachment representations of youth in residential care. *Children and Youth Services Review, 42,* 103–109. doi: 10.1016/j.childyouth.2014.04.007.

Banks, J. B., McCoy, C., & Trzcinski, C. (2018). Examining the impact of a brief human-canine interaction on stress and attention. *Human-Animal Interaction Bulletin, 6*(1), 1–13.

Banks, M. R., & Banks, W. A. (2005). The effects of group and individual animal-assisted therapy on loneliness in residents of long-term care facilities. *Anthrozoös, 18*(4), 396–408. doi: 10.2752/089279305785593983.

Bao, K. J., & Schreer, G. (2016). Pets and happiness: Examining the association between pet ownership and wellbeing. *Anthrozoös, 29*(2), 283–296. doi: 10.1080/08927936.2016.1152721.

Barak, Y., Savorai, O., Mavashev, S., & Beni, A. (2001). Animal-assisted therapy for elderly schizophrenic patients: A one-year controlled trial. *The American Journal of Geriatric Psychiatry, 9*(4), 439–442. doi: 10.1097/00019442-200111000-00013.

Barker, S. B., & Dawson, K. S. (1998). The effects of animal-assisted therapy on anxiety ratings of hospitalized psychiatric patients. *Psychiatric Services, 49*(6), 797–801.

Barker, S. B., Barker, R. T., McCain, N. L., & Schubert, C. M. (2016). A randomized cross-over exploratory study of the effect of visiting therapy dogs on college student stress before final exams. *Anthrozoös, 29*(1), 35–46. doi: 10.1080/08927936.2015.1069988.

Beetz, A. M. (2017). Theories and possible processes of action in animal assisted interventions. *Applied Developmental Science, 21*(2), 139–149. doi: 10.1080/10888691.2016.1262263.

Binfet, J. T. (2017). The effects of group-administered canine therapy on university students' wellbeing: A randomized controlled trial. *Anthrozoös, 30*(3), 397–414. doi: 10.1080/08927936.2017.1335097.

Binfet, J. T., & Passmore, H. A. (2016). Hounds and homesickness: The effects of an animal-assisted therapeutic intervention for first-year university students. *Anthrozoos, 29*, 441–454.

Braun, C., Stangler, T., Narveson, J., & Pettingell, S. (2009). Animal-assisted therapy as a pain relief intervention for children. *Complementary Therapies in Clinical Practice, 15*, 105–109.

Campbell, K., Smith, C. M., Tumilty, S., Cameron, C., & Treharne, G. J. (2016). How does dog-walking influence perceptions of health and wellbeing in healthy adults? A qualitative dog-walk-along study. *Anthrozoös, 29*(2), 181–192. doi: 10.1080/08927936.2015.1082770.

Carter, C. S., & Porges, S. W. (2016). Neural mechanisms underlying human-animal interaction: An evolutionary perspective. In L. S. Freund, S. McCune, L. Esposito, N. R. Gee, & P. McCardle (Eds.), *The social neuroscience of human-animal interaction* (pp. 89–105). Washington, DC: American Psychological Association.

Chu, C., Liu, C., Sun, C., & Lin, J. (2009). The effect of animal-assisted activity on inpatients with schizophrenia. *Journal of Psychosocial Nursing and Mental Health Services, 47*(12), 42–48. doi: 10.3928/02793695-20091103-96.

Colombo, G., Buono, M., Smania, K., Raviola, R., & De Leo, D. (2006). Pet therapy and institutionalized elderly: A study on 144 cognitively unimpaired subjects. *Archives of Gerontology and Geriatrics, 42*, 207–216.

Crossman, M. K., Kazdin, A. E., & Knudson, K. (2015). Brief unstructured interaction with a dog reduces distress. *Anthrozoos, 28*, 649–659. doi: 10.1080/08927936.2015.1070008.

Daly, B., & Suggs, S. (2010). Teachers' experiences with humane education and animals in the elementary classroom: Implications for empathy development. *Journal of Moral Education, 39*(1), 101–112. doi: 10.1080/03057240903528733.

DeLoache, J. S., Pickard, M. B., & LoBue, V. (2011). How very young children think about animals. In P. McCardle, S. McCune, J. A. Griffin, & V. Maholmes (Eds.), *How animals affect us: Examining the influences of human – animal interaction on child development and human health* (pp. 85–99). Washington, DC: American Psychological Association. doi: 10.1037/12301-004.

Epley, N., Waytz, A., & Cacioppo, J. T. (2007). On seeing human: A three-factor theory of anthropomorphism. *Psychological Review, 114*(4), 864–886. doi: 10.1037/0033-295X.114.4.86.

Evans-Wilday, A. S., Hall, S. S., Hogue, T. E., & Mills, D. S. (2018). Self-disclosure with dogs: Dog owners' and non-dog owners' willingness to disclose emotional topics. *Anthrozoös, 31*(3), 353–366. doi: 10.1080/08927936.2018.1455467.

Fine, A. H., & Gee, N. R. (2017). How animals help children learn: Introducing a roadmap for action. In N. R. Gee, A. H. Fine, & P. McCardle (Eds.), *How animals help students learn: Research and practice for educators and mental-health professionals* (pp. 3–11). New York: Routledge/Taylor & Francis Group.

Fodors. (2018). 12 North American airports where you can pet a dog. Retrieved January 22, 2019, from www.fodors.com/news/photos/12-north-american-airports-where-you-can-pet-a-therapy-dog

Gee, N. R., Church, M. T., & Altobelli, C. L. (2010). Preschoolers make fewer errors on an object categorization task in the presence of a dog. *Anthrozoös, 23*(3), 223–230. doi: 10.2752/175303710X12750451258896.

Gee, N. R., Crist, E. N., & Carr, D. N. (2010). Preschool children require fewer instructional prompts to perform a memory task in the presence of a dog. *Anthrozoös, 23*(2), 173–184. doi: 10.2752/175303710X12682332910051.

Gee, N. R., Gould, J. K., Swanson, C. C., & Wagner, A. K. (2012). Preschoolers categorize animate objects better in the presence of a dog. *Anthrozoös, 25*(2), 187–198. doi: 10.2752/175303712X13316289505387.

Grandgeorge, M., & Hausberger, M. (2011). Human-animal relationships: From daily life to animal-assisted therapies. *Annali Dell'istituto Superiore Di Sanita, 47*(4), 397–408.

Growth for Knowledge. (2018). Pet ownership. Retrieved December 17, 2018, from www.gfk.com/global-studies/global-studies-pet-ownership/

Hanselman, J. L. (2001). Coping skills interventions with adolescents in anger management using animals in therapy. *Journal of Child & Adolescent Group Therapy, 11*(4), 159–195.

Hartwig, E. K. (2017). Building solutions in youth: Evaluation of the human-animal resilience therapy intervention. *Journal of Creativity in Mental Health, 12*(4), 468–481. doi: 10.1080/15401383.2017.1283281.

Hartwig, E. K. (2019). *Animal-Assisted Counseling Academy: Frequently asked questions.* Retrieved October 10, 2018, from http://aac-academy.clas.txstate.edu/faq.html

Heinrichs, M., Baumgartner, T., Kirschbaum, C., & Ehlert, U. (2003). Social support and oxytocin interact to suppress cortisol and subjective responses to psychosocial stress. *Biological Psychiatry, 54*(12), 1389–1398.

Hergovich, A., Monshi, B., Semmler, G., & Zieglmayer, V. (2002). The effects of the presence of a dog in the classroom. *Anthrozoös, 15*(1), 37–50. doi: 10.2752/089279302786992775.

Herzog, H. (2011). The impact of pets on human health and psychological well-being: Fact, fiction, or hypothesis? *Current Directions in Psychological Science, 20*(4), 236–239. doi: 10.1177/0963721411415220.

International Association of Human-Animal Interaction Organizations. (2018). *IAHAIO white paper: The IAHAIO definitions for animal-assisted intervention and guidelines for wellness of animals involved.* Retrieved January 28, 2018, from http://iahaio.org/wp/wp-content/uploads/2018/04/iahaio_wp_updated-2018-final.pdf

Julius, H., Beetz, A., Kotrschal, K., Turner, D., & Uvnäs-Moberg, K. (2013). *Attachment to pets: An integrative view of human-animal relationships with implications for therapeutic practice.* Cambridge, MA: Hogrefe Publishing.

Krause-Parello, C. A., & Friedmann, E. (2014). The effects of an animal-assisted intervention on salivary alpha-amylase, salivary immunoglobulin A, and heart rate during forensic interviews in child sexual abuse cases. *Anthrozoös, 27*(4), 581–590. doi: 10.2752/089279314X14072268688005.

Kruger, K. A., & Serpell, J. A. (2010). Animal-assisted interventions in mental health: Definitions and theoretical foundations. In A. H. Fine (Ed.), *Handbook on animal-assisted therapy* (3rd ed., pp. 33–48). Amsterdam, The Netherlands: Elsevier. doi: 10.1016/B978-0-12-381453-1.10003-0.

Lange, A. M., Cox, J. A., Bernert, D. J., & Jenkins, C. D. (2006/2007). Is counseling going to the dogs? an exploratory study related to the inclusion of an animal in group counseling with adolescents. *Journal of Creativity in Mental Health, 2*(2), 17–31. doi: 10.1300/J456v02n02_03.

Levinson, B. (1969). *Pet-oriented child psychotherapy.* Springfield, IL: Charles C. Thomas, Bannerstone House.

Lutsky-Cohen, N., & Schneider, M. (2017). Who is interested in animal-assisted therapy (AAT)?: Features of future psychotherapists and psychologists. *Human-Animal Interaction Bulletin, 5*(2), 74–89.

Marcus, D. A., Bernstein, C. D., Constantin, J. M., Kunkel, F. A., Breuer, P., & Hanlon, R. B. (2012). Animal-assisted therapy at an outpatient pain management clinic. *Pain Medicine, 13*(1), 45–57. doi: 10.1111/j.1526-4637.2011.01294.x.

Marino, L. (2012). Construct validity of animal-assisted therapy and activities: How important is the animal in AAT? *Anthrozoös, 25*(supp 1), s139–s151. doi: 10.2752/1 75303712X13353430377219.

Martin, F., & Farnum, J. (2002). Animal-assisted therapy for children with pervasive developmental disorders. *Western Journal of Nursing Research, 24*(6), 657–670. doi: 10.1177/019394502320555403.

Mullin, M. (2002). Animals and anthropology. *Society and Animals, 10*(4), 387–394.

Nagengast, S. L., Baun, M. M., Megel, M., & Michael Leibowitz, J. (1997). The effects of the presence of a companion animal on physiological arousal and behavioral distress in children during a physical examination. *Journal of Pediatric Nursing, 12*(6), 323–330. doi: 10.1016/S0882-5963(97)80058-9.

Nimer, J., & Lundahl, B. (2007). Animal-assisted therapy: A meta-analysis. *Anthrozoos, 20*(3), 225–238. doi: 10.2752/089279307X224773.

Odendaal, J. S. J. (2000). Animal-assisted therapy – magic or medicine? *Journal of Psychosomatic Research, 49*(4), 275–280. doi: 10.1016/S0022-3999(00)00183-5.

Pendry, P., Carr, A. M., Roeter, S. M., & Vandagriff, J. L. (2018). Experimental trial demonstrates effects of animal-assisted stress prevention program on college students' positive and negative emotion. *Human-Animal Interaction Bulletin, 6*(1), 81–97.

Prothmann, A., Bienert, M., & Ettrich, C. (2006). Dogs in child psychotherapy: Effects on state of mind. *Anthrozoös, 19*(3), 265–277. doi: 10.2752/089279306785415583.

Rossetti, J., & King, C. (2010). Use of animal-assisted therapy with psychiatric patients. *Journal of Psychosocial Nursing & Mental Health Services, 48*(11), 44–48. doi: 10.3928/02793695-20100831-05.

Rud, A. G., & Beck, A. M. (2003). Companion animals in Indiana elementary schools. *Anthrozoös, 16*(3), 241–251. doi: 10.2752/089279303786992134.

Schuck, S. E. B., Emmerson, N. A., Fine, A. H., & Lakes, K. D. (2015). Canine-assisted therapy for children with ADHD. *Journal of Attention Disorders, 19*(2), 125–137. doi: 10.1177/1087054713502080.

Serpell, J., McCune, S., Gee, N., & Griffin, J. A. (2017). Current challenges to research on animal-assisted interventions. *Applied Developmental Science, 21*(3), 223–233. doi: 10.1080/10888691.2016.1262775.

Souter, M. A., & Miller, M. D. (2007). Do animal-assisted activities effectively treat depression? A meta-analysis. *Anthrozoös, 20*(2), 167–180. doi: 10.2752/1753 03707X207954.

Stefanini, M. C., Martino, A., Allori, P., Galeotti, F., & Tani, F. (2015). The use of animal-assisted therapy in adolescents with acute mental disorders: A randomized controlled study. *Complementary Therapies in Clinical Practice, 21*(1), 42–46. doi: 10.1016/j.ctcp.2015.01.001.

Tsai, C. C., Friedmann, E., & Thomas, S. A. (2010). The effect of animal-assisted therapy on stress responses in hospitalized children. *Anthrozoos, 23*, 245–258.

Ward-Griffin, E., Klaiber, P., Collins, H. K., Owens, R. L., Coren, S., & Chen, F. S. (2018). Petting away pre-exam stress: The effect of therapy dog sessions on student well-being. *Stress and Health, 34*, 468–473. doi: 10.1002/smi.2804.

Wilson, E. O. (1984). *Biophilia*. Cambridge, MA: Harvard University Press.

Wood, L. J. (2011). Community benefits of human-animal interactions: The ripple effect. In P. McCardle, S. McCune, J. A. Griffin, L. Esposito, & L. S. Freund (Eds.), *Animals in our lives: Human – animal interaction in family, community, and therapeutic settings* (pp. 23–42). Baltimore, MD: Paul H Brookes Publishing.

Zilcha-Mano, S., Mikulincer, M., & Shaver, P. R. (2011). Pet in the therapy room: An attachment perspective on animal-assisted therapy. *Attachment & Human Development, 13*(6), 541–561. doi: 10.1080/14616734.2011.608987.

3 What Makes a Strong and Effective Canine-Assisted Intervention Team?

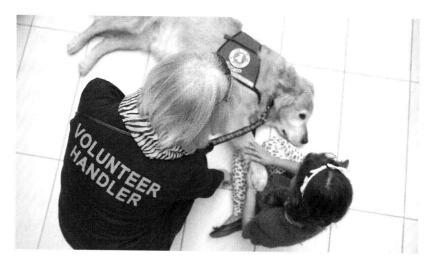

Figure 3.1 Volunteer handler Moira facilitates an interaction between her dog and a visiting child.

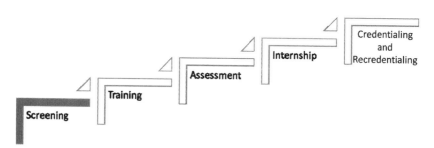

Figure 3.2 CAI team credentialing process.

The aim of this chapter is to provide readers with information on the characteristics and dispositions of strong CAI teams. In this chapter we provide an overview of the skills needed by teams and lay the foundation for the credentialing process just introduced in Chapter 1.

Scenario

> Recently divorced and looking to fill a void in her life, Susan adopted a dog from her local shelter. Not wanting the work entailed in raising a puppy, Susan opted for a 3-year-old mixed-breed Labrador she called William. Her new dog got her out of the house, allowing her to meet new people. In fact, it was William who seemed to facilitate most of the introductions! On walks William ignored other dogs and, at every chance, gravitated to people. He'd nuzzle in, roll on his back, seeking tummy rubs, and loved to lean into people to keep close. Susan repeatedly heard, "This dog should be a therapy dog!" Having no experience with therapy dogs, and with herself in therapy to deal with issues arising from her divorce, Susan wondered, "What does it take to get into a therapy dog program, and should I be trying to help others when I myself need help?"

Questions for Reflection and Discussion

1. Can rescue dogs make good therapy dogs? If so, do they require extra screening and scrutiny?
2. In urban centers where multiple CAI organizations operate, what distinguishes a strong from a mediocre organization?
3. Is being a CAI handler therapeutic for the handler too?

The previous scenario raises a number of issues around just how to identify the qualities of both a strong handler and therapy dog—the CAI team. Throughout this chapter, we emphasize the team dynamic that captures a handler and dog working in unison. Having just reviewed the different categories of CAIs and the pathways to supporting well-being across a variety of contexts in the previous chapter, we'll now explore the foundational skills needed by CAI teams for participation in CAIs.

CAI Organizations

Recall that one of our primary aims in writing this book is to reduce some of the variability in the screening, training, and assessment of CAI teams. Certainly, one source of the variability we see in current screening practices lies in the variability of CAI organizations themselves. There is currently no comprehensive list of CAI organizations in operation around the world. In our review of therapy dog organizations with active websites, we identified 320 organizations in just the United States and Canada alone (Hartwig & Binfet, 2019). A cursory review of web-based listings of therapy dog organizations reveals a variety of iterations (i.e., from international organizations to home-grown programs) operating in virtually every developed country.

There are thus numerous national and international organizations that support hundreds of local animal therapy organizations throughout the world. With the combination of both large-scale and independently run organizations, it's easy to see how challenging it can be for there to be consistency across organizations around the screening, training, and assessing of CAI teams. Additionally, the laws, values, and perceptions about therapy dogs differ across nations and even by regions within a country. For these reasons, the CAI field has been challenged in developing standardized criteria. Our focus in this chapter is to identify the foundational prerequisites that can be employed by CAI organizations across contexts to identify strong CAI teams who will represent them well in their work to support human well-being.

The Importance of Published Criteria

An important step for CAI organizations is that criteria be published online and in print for prospective CAI teams. If potential handlers don't know what the requirements are to become a CAI team, how can they decide to pursue this opportunity? In our in-depth review of 64 randomly selected CAI organizations from over 320 organizations identified in the United States and Canada, we found no established standardized, shared criteria for CAI programs (Hartwig & Binfet, 2019). The variability in our findings is consistent with the lack of governance in the CAI field across a multitude of independent CAI organizations in operation. Members of the public who are considering investing their time and energy to become a credentialed CAI team should be fully aware of required training, assessment, and expectations around the ongoing monitoring of teams once they're credentialed. As we argue in Chapter 8, it is important that CAI organizations combine their use of standardized screening, training, and assessment practices with nuanced screening, training, and assessment practices that prepare CAI teams for work with distinctive populations and contexts served by the CAI organization.

Understanding Trends in Volunteering

Although some CAI organizations have a director-level position that is salaried, the majority of the work done on behalf of a CAI organization is done by volunteers. Understanding the science behind volunteering helps inform organization personnel around how best to identify volunteers and what to expect from volunteers over time, once they have been selected for participation in a program. It's important to note too that there are many teams who work in professional settings providing canine-assisted therapy (CAT) or canine-assisted counseling (CAC). Within these contexts, the handler is a trained professional and not a volunteer. Thus, for the purposes of our book, we make a clear distinction between CAI teams who volunteer on behalf of a CAI organization and practitioners who incorporate CAIs as part of the professional services they offer to clients. As our focus in this chapter is on CAI volunteer teams, we'll explore trends in volunteering that might inform our understanding of CAI teams volunteering on behalf of a CAI organization.

There are a few key findings found across studies on volunteering that might help shed light on the volunteer dog-handler profile. First, across all age groups

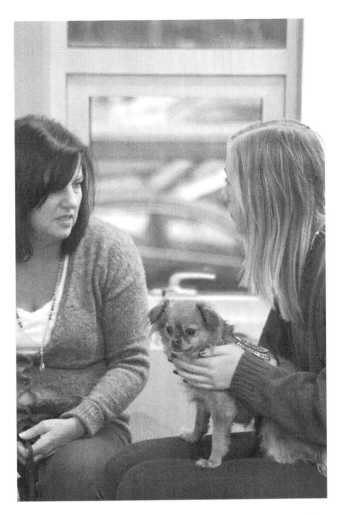

Figure 3.3 Volunteer handler Colleen and her dog, Monkey, support a college student.

and educational levels, women tend to volunteer more than men (U.S. Bureau of Labor Statistics, 2013). Second, people who are married volunteer at a higher rate than do unmarried individuals. Third, most volunteers restrict their volunteer service to just one or two organizations. Last, there appears to be a declining trend in the rate of volunteering (i.e., fewer people are volunteering over time). In a recent publication on volunteering, Hyde and colleagues (2014) posit that the declining volunteer rate may be due to the increased time constraints we face or to the trend toward participating in "episodic volunteering"—volunteer opportunities that do not require a sustained commitment over time and may be a one-off or short-term volunteer experience. In light of the resources that CAI organizations invest in screening and selecting teams, CAI organization personnel would be wise to keep abreast of findings in the broader field of volunteering as a means of honing their ability to identify reliable and long-term volunteers to work on their behalf.

CAI Organization Variability

Before we delve into the characteristics or qualities that make strong CAI teams, an overview of CAI organizations in general is warranted. As we mentioned, the scale of CAI organizations varies, and although there are a few national-level organizations, in our recent review of CAI organizations, we identified that the bulk of organizations operate at the local or regional levels (Hartwig & Binfet, 2019). What this means is that individuals within a community who have an interest in therapy dogs and community well-being coalesce resources to procure funding and liability insurance; establish community connections; screen, train, and assess CAI teams; and hopefully monitor the ongoing delivery of services to community members.

On the horizon we suspect, at the time of our writing, there are no universally accepted and adhered-to standards for the screening, training, and assessment of therapy dogs for participation in community-based well-being initiatives. Added to this, there is ample variability in the training, background, and formation of the personnel who oversee individual CAI organizations, and as a consequence, there is also variability in the processes used to identify CAI teams. As a result, the skills and competencies of CAI teams chosen and subsequently credentialed for participation in CAI organizations varies considerably.

As an illustration of how this variability plays out in the field, consider briefly a local CAI organization whose mandate has largely been to provide support to geriatric patients at a retirement facility. As interest in CAI organizations has grown, this group, the only group in the city, has been asked to provide therapy dogs to reduce stress in employees at a 911 emergency call center. Are therapy dogs who are accustomed to working with a relatively quiet client group within a controlled environment such as a retirement home well suited to working with multiple, varied-age clients within a busy context where employees are known to have elevated stress levels? Once an organization has credentialed CAI teams, does this mean these teams are suited to working with any client group within any setting? We argue in the following sections and in Chapter 8 that nuanced screening, training, and assessment of CAI teams is required—certainly in light of the demand for therapy dogs to support the well-being of varied clients in varied settings.

Best Practices of CAI Organizations

Little has been written on the characteristics of the CAI organization as an entity in and of itself as the focus has predominantly been on the assessment of dogs and, to a lesser extent, on identifying suitable handlers. Linder and colleagues (2017) conducted a national survey of the health and safety policies in animal therapy organizations. Though restricted by the small sample size (i.e., only 27 organizations) used in this study, their findings confirm that there is ample variability in both the policies and practices of animal therapy organizations. Using an online survey approach to glean information about each organization, these researchers asked questions about the "organization's policies on animal health status and records, types of animals permitted in the program, and obedience testing criteria" (Linder, Siebens, Mueller, Gibbs, & Freeman, 2017, p. 884). Their findings revealed variations in the health screenings required by organizations (e.g., in asking for rabies vaccines or fecal test results) and also in the behavioral requirements necessary for assessing therapy canines. For example, one-third of the organizations surveyed relied *uniquely* on the American Kennel Club (AKC, 2019) Canine Good Citizen certificate—a certificate Linder and colleagues (2017) acknowledge is not designed to assess suitability for CAI work. The findings of this study are in alignment with what we've previously argued in Chapter 1 and earlier in this chapter: notably, that there is variability in the training or expertise of the individuals overseeing CAI organizations and variability in the screening, training, assessment, and day-to-day operations that guide program delivery.

In an effort to identify the policies of CAI organizations that uphold best practices, we now turn our attention to the gold-standard characteristics of organizations that provide the pubic with access to therapy dogs. As a starting point and a point of reference, the AKC identifies seven characteristics they use to help screen CAI organizations in an effort to determine organizations worthy of their endorsement (AKC, 2019). For inclusion in the AKC list of recognized CAI organizations, the following criteria must be met: (1) groups are nonprofits (i.e., 501(c)3), (2) operate under the guidance of a board of directors, (3) have experienced therapy dog handlers working with them who have been certified, (4) have individual liability insurance policies for each handler-dog team, (5) have their own therapy-specific assessment, (6) have an established track record of at least 1 year working with facilities, and (7) have a training program for handlers.

In addition to these characteristics, well-run CAI organizations should also include the following practices as part of their day-to-day operations:

1. Make information available regarding their training and assessment and the qualifications of the program's leadership, directors, and evaluators.
2. Have a published and clearly articulated mission or vision statement that reflects the purpose, aims, and philosophy of the program.
3. Use evidence-based best practices in screening, training, and assessing CAI teams that includes the use of multiple assessors or raters.
4. Monitor and supervise CAI teams working on behalf of the organization out in the field and provide routine formative feedback to strengthen their skills.

5. Where diverse clients are served, ensure CAI teams are trained and assessed for specific clients and specific contexts.
6. Provide professional development opportunities for handlers once teams have been credentialed.
7. Offer recredentialing of CAI teams post-initial assessment, recognizing that dogs' behavior and dispositions can change over time.
8. Keep track of all documentation (e.g., vaccine records, criminal record background check for handlers) for, and service done by, individual CAI teams.
9. Work in partnership with a veterinarian or veterinary clinic who advises on best practices for optimal canine welfare and health within programs.
10. Operate in the spirit of transparency and publishes a year-end report that includes number of handlers, types and number of sessions and programs offered, number of volunteer hours completed by handlers, number of clients served, a safety record, and financial support received.

Publishing CAI Team Prerequisites and Criteria

In this section we'll review prerequisite criteria that CAI organizations should publish online and request as part of the application process. As mentioned previously, publishing criteria allows potential handlers to assess if the volunteer opportunity is a good fit for them and their dogs. The organization's published criteria should also match the information requested on the handler-screening application. For example, if an organization requires that a dog be at least 1 year old, then the application should request the age of the dog. In this instance, there is no need for organization personnel to review applications of handlers with dogs who are still puppies.

Additionally, organizations should be specific about the client populations they serve, as a CAI team may be a better fit for working with certain populations (e.g., children, seniors, college students, travelers, people in crisis).

Determining Initial Suitability of Handlers

After several years running our own CAI organizations and research studies, we have learned that before investing time, energy, and resources into a potential CAI team, we should address the feasibility of a handler team's involvement by asking the following two questions:

1. Does the handler's schedule allow for participation in the programs scheduled by the organization?
2. Does the handler live within a reasonable geographic area that would allow for easy access to program sites?

As our CAI programs are offered at various times during the day (e.g., from a morning program at the local police precinct to an after-school program for local children) handlers who work full-time, 9 a.m. to 5 p.m., in jobs with little flexibility are not a match for the work we do. As such, there is no sense in screening handlers and assessing the dogs of handlers who cannot be available at the times our programs are offered. Assessing a strong CAI team only to find out they cannot support the program because of a scheduling conflict amounts to a waste of resources.

Related to this, our other initial screening question is to ask whether potential handlers live within a reasonable geographic distance from our program sites. It is disappointing to have a dog/handler team scheduled and have them cancel because of poor road conditions or traffic delays. We typically book two to three extra dogs for sessions as we find handlers adjusting their schedules or unable to attend because their dogs are not well or they themselves are under the weather. As such, and even with extra dogs booked, we occasionally put a short-notice call out for a substitute dog/handler team and having handlers live nearby program sites has made finding substitute handlers easy.

As a means of reducing office resources devoted to screening potential CAI teams, organizations can create a CAI Team Screening Form that puts the onus on the handler to provide information that helps them determine suitability and asks the two previous questions (regarding scheduling and location of residence) to help organizations narrow their search for candidates who hold the most potential to be strong handlers within the organization. This is in alignment with protocols followed by the larger CAI organizations who typically have an online initial information form for prospective CAI teams to complete or have potential handlers watch a webinar as an initial first step (e.g., Pet Partners). In contrast, some of the smaller CAI organizations use a phone call interview to screen potential handlers (e.g., Paws & Hearts of Palm Springs, CA; Paws & Hearts, 2019). Regardless of the means through which handlers are initially screened, taking steps to ascertain the suitability of a potential handler for a program helps avoid investing resources in assessing CAI teams who, in the end, are not an ideal fit.

CAI Team Screening Form

In this section we'll discuss information that should be requested of CAI teams as part of an initial screening process. This information can be addressed in a paper or online form, or even though an interview with a potential handler. We will discuss the following screening form topics: basic information, motivation to volunteer, relationship, temperament, experience, experience with animals, training, background check, equipment, and availability. A sample CAI Team Screening Form is available in **Appendix A** at the end of the book.

Basic Information

This information allows a CAI organization to know who is applying to be a volunteer handler and how to contact them. Some organizations have minimum age requirements, such as the requirement for a handler to be at least 18 years of age; therefore, it's important to ask for an applicant's date of birth or about meeting the established minimum age requirements. Basic information about the dog is also collected at this point and provides the organization with information that will help identify the dog during training and assessments.

What to address for this topic:

- *Handler:* Name, address, phone number, e-mail address, and date of birth
- *Dog:* Name, date of birth or age, breed, and spay/neuter status

Motivation to Volunteer

Both handlers and dogs should be suited for CAI work with specific populations. It's important to explore why potential handlers would like to volunteer on behalf of the organization and with the population they serve, as well as how the dog might respond to working with the population.

What to address for this topic:

- *Handler:* Why a person wants to volunteer with the organization and the population served by the organization
- *Dog:* How the dog might respond to working with the organization or population served by the organization

Relationship

One of the most important things to assess in a potential team is the relationship between the handler and her or his dog. Asking handlers to reflect on this on the application gives the CAI organization initial insight into how the handler and dog work together.

What to address for this topic:

- *Handler:* The human-canine relationship
- *Dog:* How the handler and dog function as a team

Temperament

Handlers should be friendly, enjoy interacting with the populations served by the organization, and willing to put in the time and effort to become a credentialed CAI team.

What to address for this topic:

- *Handler:* A handler's temperament, personality, and ability to connect with others
- *Dog:* Additional information about a dog's temperament and behavior when meeting new people and explore how the dog responds to different people

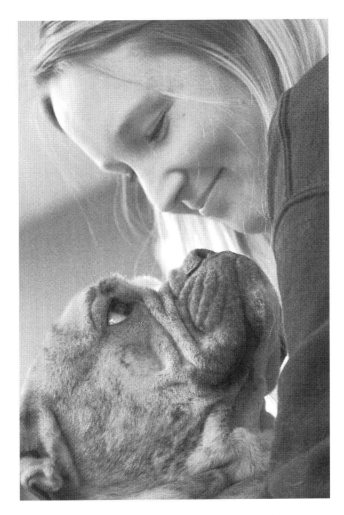

Figure 3.4 Volunteer handler Kristina and her therapy dog, Tugboat.

Experience

Previous volunteer or work experience with the target population demonstrates an interest, knowledge about, and ability to work with potential clients (e.g., day care or camp counselor experience with children demonstrates that the handler has already worked with children). For the dog, has dog ever volunteered with another agency? Has the dog been trained for other public work? Also consider the dog's time with the handler. Has the handler had sufficient time to see the dog interact with people, learn the dog's patterns and behavior, and observe if the dog has challenges or hesitancies when interacting with people or in certain situations?

What to address for this topic:

- *Handler*: Any relevant volunteer or work experience, as well as experience with potential populations (seniors, children, hospitals)
- *Dog*: Any relevant volunteer or work experience and time with the handler

Experience With Animals

It's important to assess if handlers and dogs have had positive and negative experiences around other animals. For handlers, positive experiences with animals show that the handler enjoys interacting with animals. Negative experiences show any potential fears or issues the handler may have around dogs or other animals (e.g., if the handler was bitten by a dog as a child, the handler may be anxious around CAI teams with dogs resembling the dog from their childhood experience). If the dog has had a previous negative experience with certain people (e.g., children, men) or situations (e.g., loud noises), the dog may respond unpredictably if exposed to similar people or situations.

What to address for this topic:

- *Handler*: Positive or negative experiences with animals
- *Dog*: Positive or negative experiences with people and other animals

Training

It is important to explore handlers' values and beliefs about training and the training experience. Equally important is to understand the dog's training history.

What to address for this topic:

- *Handler*: Training with the dog, including location, type of training (puppy, intermediate, agility, Canine Good Citizen, tricks), trainer, trainer credentials
- *Dog*: Registrations or certifications, working dog training

Background Check

The handlers who work with specific populations (e.g., children, vulnerable clients) must have a clear criminal background in order to work with vulnerable populations. Depending on the resources of the CAI organization, handlers may be required to pay this fee themselves. It's also important to understand each dog's history of aggression as a means to identifying dogs who are a poor fit for therapy work.

What to address for this topic:

- *Handler:* No criminal history or allegations; a fingerprint check as part of the criminal background check is key for vulnerable populations
- *Dog:* No history of aggression with people or other animals

Equipment

Knowing which training equipment handlers use is important, as it can be helpful in assessing the handler-dog relationship and the dog's behavioral profile. This includes asking handlers which collars (e.g., has the dog been exposed to training with collars that are aversive or corrective, such as prong collars or e-collars?) and leash (e.g., has dog only walked on a retractable leash?) have been used in training the dog.

What to address for this topic:

- *Handler:* The training equipment used by handlers
- *Dog:* Type of collar and leash

Availability

This information allows your organization to know the availability of potential handlers. Programs run at specific times, and thus, knowledge of availability to participate in various sessions is helpful. Some organizations have minimum participation requirements or may be looking for handlers to participate in programs offered during specific timeslots.

What to address for this topic:

- *Handler and Dog:* Which day(s) and times is the team available each week

The full CAI Team Screening Form can be found in **Appendix A**.

The CAI Team

When reviewing the screening, training, and assessment criteria for having a pet dog credentialed as a therapy dog by a local CAI organization, it is evident that the emphasis has historically been on assessing characteristics of the dog. This was clear in our aforementioned study on the screening criteria used by CAI organizations, who, for the most part, focused on characteristics of the dog while largely overlooking the importance of screening handlers and of the team component necessary for successful work in CAI organizations (Hartwig & Binfet, 2019). In the following sections we review the behaviors, skills, and dispositions required of handlers for successful participation in CAIs.

Handler's Commitment to Maintaining Hygiene

A prospective handler seeking to become credentialed along with her or his dog as a CAI team should adhere to exemplary standards of hygiene from the moment he or she establishes contact with the CAI organization—whether that be at a handler-only orientation session to learn information about becoming credentialed or at an assessment where prospective CAI teams are evaluated on a series of behaviors and dispositions. The template for a Canine Health Screening Form is provided in **Appendix B**.

Handler Hygiene

Handlers are encouraged to restrict their use of heavy colognes or perfumes, as these can both challenge a dog's intense sense of smell and prove problematic in facilities that are declared scent-free.

Canine Hygiene

Dogs should be bathed and brushed prior to participating in training or assessment sessions. Handlers may think of training as a practice time for their upcoming work in their role as a CAI team member. If a dog smells, has matted fur, or open wounds, a message is conveyed to clients and the community that the dog's hygiene and health are not a priority.

Canine Health

Dogs should also have up-to-date vaccines, including rabies (many organizations will ask that a copy of the rabies certificate be brought to the first training session), and be on a flea preventative to prohibit the spreading of fleas to other dogs in attendance, should fleas be prevalent in the area. If a dog exhibits any signs of sickness, such as diarrhea, vomiting, or lethargy, the training appointment should be canceled, as should all program sessions once the CAI team is credentialed. In addition to maintaining a vaccine regimen, handlers are asked to maintain a deworming regimen to safeguard against their dog harboring parasites.

Canine Diet

There is much discussion within CAI organization circles about diet and in particular around therapy dogs being fed a raw diet as doing so is commonly thought to increase the chance of dog-to-human zoonotic disease (Lefebre, Reid-Smith, Boerlin, & Weese, 2008). One theme throughout our book has been to showcase the variability in the CAI field and when it comes to the diet of therapy dogs, there is certainly ample variability in best practice recommendations.

Our recommendation regarding diet is for CAI organizations to develop a protocol in consultation with their veterinarian and to establish guidelines for CAI teams in light of the client population they serve.

Handler Disposition

As CAI organizations seek new handlers, one overriding dimension for which handlers should be screened is that handlers should embrace the qualities they're seeking to support in clients. As a simple illustration of this, if a handler is working in an on-campus stress-reduction program for college students, the handler should not be characterized by high stress and moreover should have coping mechanisms in place and put into practice that keep their stress in check. Similarly, if a handler is assigned to support groups of elderly residents in a retirement facility who are known to feel lonely and isolated, the handler must have strong interpersonal social and emotional skills that can be used to encourage interactions with the therapy dog and interactions among residents to build community. Thus, undergirding the selection of handlers is the recognition of the handler embodying the very characteristics they are trying to support in clients.

Canine Temperament and Skills

Susan, the dog owner in our opening scenario, repeatedly heard that her dog William would make a great therapy dog. On the surface, William's interest in greeting strangers and calm behavior in public are certainly strong indicators that he might very well make a strong therapy dog; however, much more needs to be discovered about William's temperament and ability to work with the public. Fredrickson-MacNamara and Butler (2010, p. 126) describe the challenge for therapy dogs as follows: "The key is in determining whether an animal has the capacity to recover from the encroachment of strangers, cope comfortably in the environment, and respond appropriately to interactions."

What Is Asked of a Therapy Dog?

Before identifying the ideal traits or desired characteristics of therapy dogs, it is important to acknowledge just what is asked of therapy dogs. First, therapy dogs are asked to work in public spaces. What is known about public spaces, whether it be the recreation room of a retirement facility or the departure level of an airport, is that unanticipated and novel stimuli are commonplace. This might include the passing of a noisy janitorial cart, the dropping of food by folks passing by, or loud noises.

Second, though the target client in need of support may well be identified, when working in a public setting, therapy dogs often attract the enthusiastic attention of the general public. This might include a toddler who breaks free from his mother's grasp and runs over to the dogs, schoolchildren on a field trip who can't hold back their excitement at seeing the dogs, or adults working in the building who themselves are curious to learn more about why the dogs are present. Therapy dogs working in public spaces may also encounter people who are fearful of dogs, have limited experience with dogs, or have cultural views of dogs that are not in alignment with the views shared by the CAI organization. A further complication arises when therapy dogs who are working in public settings encounter someone out for a walk with their dog and who insist on bringing their dog over to greet the therapy dogs. The potential for interdog conflict arises in such situations, and visits by public dogs shift the therapy dog's attention from being human focused to fellow dog focused.

Last, increasingly, we see a trend in which multiple therapy dogs are brought to a public location to provide support to clients. This is done largely to meet the demand and interest of the clients, as a one-on-one approach would be too time consuming and would leave clients waiting and potentially frustrated. Certainly, we see this model of multiple dogs used in CAI programs on college campuses. This, in turn, requires therapy dogs to have strong interdog compatibility yet remain human focused in the presence of other dogs. This is akin to a person being at a party or social gathering but not being allowed to talk to anyone. Reviewing the complexities of the challenges presented to therapy dogs working in public spaces, we see that a lot is asked of them. Next, we'll delve into the specific characteristics of therapy dogs that help safeguard public safety and provide optimal support to clients.

Assessing Therapy Dogs

In Chapter 7 we will explore, in depth, just how the CAI team can be assessed and subsequently credentialed for participation in CAIs. Here, we discuss in broad terms the behaviors and dispositions needed by therapy dogs. Keep in mind the primary rationale for screening, training, and assessing therapy dogs—to ensure that dogs working in public spaces to support human well-being have sound temperament and behavior and present no danger to the public (Binfet & Struik, 2018).

Can Rescue Dogs Make Good Therapy Dogs?

Stereotypically, when asked to describe a therapy dog, the public would likely identify golden retrievers, Labrador retrievers, and perhaps poodles. As the field of CAI grows, so, too, does the diversity in dog breeds seen working in CAI organizations to support human well-being. Certainly, the aforementioned dog breeds remain popular staples in the CAI world; however, increasingly, we see mixed-breed dogs participating in CAIs.

The experience of William, the Lab cross in our opening scenario, illustrates a typical trajectory for some of these mixed-breed dogs; adopted from a shelter, once settled in his new home, he displays characteristics and dispositions that even the public deem suitable for therapy work. Readers curious

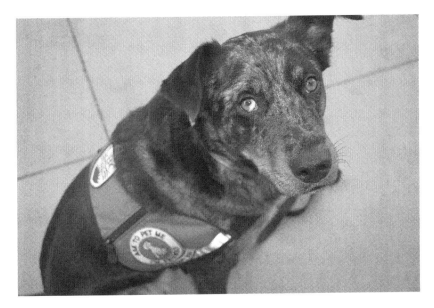

Figure 3.5 Therapy dog Frances from UBC's B.A.R.K. program.

about this topic are encouraged to search images for therapy dogs on Google Images—what you'll see is, not surprisingly, ample images of golden retrievers; however, you'll also see several mixed-breed dogs represented.

Behavioral Indicators

Delving more deeply into the characteristics of dogs that render them suitable for CAIs, we now explore canine behavioral indicators that help identify therapy dog suitability. Jones and Gosling (2005), in their comprehensive review of canine personality and temperament, identified the following seven standard behavioral dimensions or indicators: (1) reactivity, (2) fearfulness, (3) activity level, (4) sociability, (5) responsiveness to training, (6) submissiveness, and (7) problem behaviors. These behavioral dimensions certainly can serve as a foundation to guide the evaluation of potential therapy dogs, but more nuanced indicators of a dog's suitability to do therapeutic work are needed.

Basic Canine Skills

In our opening scenario, shelter dog William demonstrated skills that, according to the people he met out on walks, rendered him a strong candidate for work as a therapy dog. Initial impressions of a dog's skills are important;

however, a more careful examination of basic canine skills is needed. Successful therapy dogs must demonstrate the following behavior and dispositions.

Advanced Canine Therapeutic Skills

With time, experience, and guidance, therapy dogs can learn and demonstrate advanced behaviors that enhance their interactions with clients and visitors. This can include (1) leaning into clients when clients are seated; (2) holding positions that invite and encourage interactions, such as rolling upside down to allow a belly rub; (3) resting their head on the shoulder of a client to show affection; (4) working in varied settings; and (5) working with a variety of clients.

As an illustration of these advanced skills, the Building Academic Retention Through K9s (B.A.R.K.) program at the University of British Columbia expanded its programming beyond the stress-reduction sessions it typically offers for students on campus. Approached by the superintendent of the local police detachment, B.A.R.K. was asked to provide therapy dogs to reduce police officer stress within the local precinct on a weekly basis. In addition to the advanced screening by handers required (i.e., advanced background security checks), dogs were required to demonstrate advanced skills that included passing through a security door, riding an elevator with other dogs, working in proximity to other therapy dogs, interacting with uniformed police officers, and adjusting to the smell of firearms.

Table 3.1 Basic Skills and Behaviors Required of Therapy Dogs

Skill	Behaviors
Basic obedience	The ability to respond with high compliance to the handler's requests to sit, stay, leave it, and down
Secure attachment	To be securely attached to handlers and not demonstrate behaviors indicating insecurity (e.g., hiding behind the handler, seeking comfort from the handler when approached)
Calm behavior in public	To demonstrate a high startle reflex, as many therapy dogs work in busy settings; that is, they must not be easily startled and should have a calm public disposition
Focus	To be human focused and not focused on interacting with other dogs in the vicinity
Approachability and acceptance of touch	The ability to accept being approached by strangers and not show signs of cowering or fear-based reactions (e.g., seeking comfort from the handler).
Interest in meeting new people	At the core, to show interest in meeting new people and in interacting with the public; "Does the dog want to do this work?" is a guiding question during the screening and selection process
Interdog compatibility	As several therapy dogs may work side by side within the same area, to show no aggression when multiple dogs are present

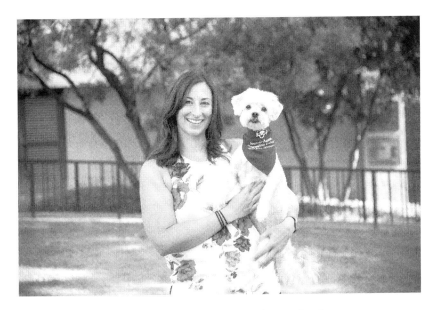

Figure 3.6 CAC practitioner Leah Walter and her therapy dog, Junior.

Once a CAI team is credentialed by an organization, there doesn't yet appear to be a stratified structure in place within organizations to recognize a team's level of expertise. That said, the American Kennel Club (AKC, 2019), as part of its Therapy Dog Program subdivision (see www.akc.org/sports/title-recogni tion-program/therapy-dog-program/) acknowledges differences in experience by awarding *novice* to *distinguished* AKC Therapy Dog titles. Their overriding criterion is the number of visits earned by the dog/handler team, with 10 visits awarded a novice title whereas 400 visits or more are required for the distinguished title. In order to have an AKC title bestowed upon a CAI team, the team must be certified by an AKC-recognized therapy dog organization.

Handler Skills

As mentioned earlier in this chapter, the focus of the assessment of CAI teams has predominantly been on the skills required of therapy dogs with little mention of the skills required by handlers. There is, however, initial work by Fredrickson-MacNamara and Butler (2010, p. 127) that was adapted by Binfet and Struik (2018, p. 21) recognizing the importance of handler skills during canine visitation. These include the following:

1.   Demonstrate appropriate treatment of people and animals.
2.   Demonstrate social skills (e.g., eye contact, smiles, confident posture, conversation) that engage people in the AAIs.

3. Prepare for, conduct, and conclude a visit.
4. Demonstrate handling methods that help participants attain their target goals.
5. Respect and maintain confidentiality.
6. Demonstrate pleasant, calm, and friendly reaction to, and attitude toward, animals during sessions.
7. Demonstrate proactive (rather than reactive) animal handling skills.
8. Act as the animal's advocate during sessions, protecting and respecting the animal's needs.
9. Effectively interpret the animal's cues (i.e., stress, excitement) and respond accordingly.

It goes without saying that the handler plays an especially important role within the CAI team. The handler must juggle overseeing and managing her or his dog while meeting the needs of clients. We recommend the following basic or standard skills be required of handlers.

Dog Handling Skills:

*   positioning the dog to facilitate client access (e.g., optimizing access to the dog for clients to encourage interaction/contact)
*   monitoring canine stress and well-being (e.g., recognizing canine stress indicators, monitoring length of session)
*   safeguarding canine welfare (e.g., redirecting inappropriate petting or roughhousing with canines, preventing clients from feeding dogs unless directed)

Human Interaction Skills:

*   demonstrating strong social and emotional skills when engaging with clients (e.g., strong empathic listening)
*   practicing perspective taking so that the handler is able to put him- or herself into the shoes of the client and understand her or his emotional world; this is especially important in stress-reduction programs that serve populations known to experience heightened stress
*   encouraging interactions between the dog and client (e.g., inviting and encouraging hands-on contact with the dog)
*   recognizing and referring clients who require additional support to additional outside resources in accordance with program policy and protocol
*   being an ambassador for the CAI organization (e.g., sharing information about the program that might include its mission, dates of upcoming events, etc.)

Both handlers and therapy dogs need strong social skills for interacting with clients.

The Importance of Interpreting Canine Behavior

The training of prospective CAI teams for assessment leading to credentialing by a CAI organization should include a component that teaches handlers how to interpret canine behavior—both behavior that indicates the dog is in distress and behavior that indicates the dog is relaxed and enjoying the session. Training by the CAI organization can make use of visuals to illustrate to handlers examples of such signs, and there are ample examples to be found on video-sharing platforms such as YouTube.

The Importance of Mock, Real-World, and Multiple-Skill Assessments

After the initial behavioral screening, training, and assessment to identify potential CAI teams, it is important that skills be assessed both in mock and real-world settings to evaluate the extent the skills that were displayed in isolation have transferability to real-world, applied settings where a number of complexities come into play. In social science research this is referred to as *ecological validity*, and it is an important consideration when investigating how skills or behaviors evident in a controlled setting come to life in a real-world context.

Practice Assessments

Practice assessments involve introducing stimuli and re-creating a setting that mirrors what would be encountered when the CAI team participates in the CAI assessment and then later is sent out to work on behalf of an organization. Practice assessments might involve borrowing a wheelchair and having a volunteer in a wheelchair approach a dog to gauge her or his reaction. The rationale here is that the dog's reaction to the wheelchair would provide an indication of how the dog might react when a client in a wheelchair, perhaps even a motorized wheelchair, approaches a CAI station out in public.

Practice assessments are especially useful for identifying aversive reactions by dogs. For example, in a practice assessment, a therapy dog candidate could be introduced to people with varied skin tones and people wearing varied clothing (e.g., hats or a headwrap). As dogs can react differently to people with darkly pigmented skin (Coren, 2016) and are known to use their owner's reaction to new people as a reference point to inform their own reaction (Duranton, Bedossa, & Gaunet, 2016), a practice session in which dogs' reactions to new and diverse individuals are assessed within a safe context is preferable to having a strong, potentially aggressive reaction in a public setting. The same scenario holds for the assessment of candidate dogs for work with young children. We will discuss this further in Chapter 8 when we discuss the requirements of CAI teams working in reading programs in public schools.

Internship

It is recommended that new CAI teams be accepted by an organization pending the successful completion of a conditional internship within a real-world setting. Under the supervision and tutelage of a program director or an experienced CAI handler or supervisor who mentors new handlers, new CAI teams can have their behavior corrected, shaped, or encouraged to meet the needs and goals of the organization. It is during this internship that handler skills are especially malleable and that it is understood that this is a time when handlers are still learning the nuanced skills needed for having their dog work in public. This might include reminders about positioning the dog so that he or she is accessible to clients, avoiding interactions with other dogs working in the vicinity, or being more socially and emotionally engaged with clients during sessions.

Conclusion

The aim of this chapter was to introduce readers to the broad skills required of both handlers and therapy dogs for successful work in varied well-being community-based initiatives. Given the public nature of the work required by CAI teams supporting CAI well-being initiatives, the screening, training, and assessment of both dogs and their handlers is of utmost importance in ensuring public safety. CAI organizations who take the time to ensure CAI teams are thoughtfully and comprehensively screened, trained, and assessed can have handlers who serve as exemplary ambassadors for their organization all the while providing support to community members seeking comfort through interactions with therapy dogs.

References

American Kennel Club. (AKC). (2019). AKC *recognized therapy dog organizations.* Retrieved from https://www.akc.org/sports/title-recognition-program/therapy-dog-program/therapy-dog-organizations/

Binfet, J. T., & Struik, K. (2018). Dogs on campus: Holistic assessment of therapy dogs and handlers for research and community initiatives. *Society & Animals: Journal of Human-Animal Studies.* Retrieved from https://brill.com/downloadpdf/journals/soan/. . ./article-10.1163-15685306-12341495.pdf

Bureau of Labor Statistics, U.S. Department of Labor (2013). Volunteering in the United States –2013. Retrieved from www.bls.gov/news.release/archives/volun_0225 2014.pdf

Coren, S. (2016, February 10). Is it possible that a dog could be racist? *Psychology Today.* Retrieved from www.psychologytoday.com/us/blog/canine-corner/201602/is-it-possible-dog-could-be-racist

Duranton, C., Bedossa, T., & Gaunet, F. (2016). When facing an unfamiliar person, pet dogs present social referencing based on their owner's direction of movement alone. *Animal Behaviour, 113,* 147–156.

Fredrickson-MacNamara, M., & Butler, K. (2010). Animal selection procedures in animal-assisted interaction programs. In A. H. Fine (Ed.), *Handbook on animal-assisted therapy: Theoretical foundations and guidelines for practice* (3rd ed., pp. 111–134). New York: Academic Press.

Hartwig, E. K., & Binfet, J. T. (2019). What's important in canine-assisted intervention teams? An investigation of canine-assisted intervention program online screening tools. *Journal of Veterinary Behavior: Clinical Applications and Research, 29,* 53–60.

Hyde, M. K., Dunn, J., Scuffham, P. A., & Chambers, S. K. (2014). A systematic review of episodic volunteering in public health and other contexts. *BMC Public Health, 14,* 992–1008. doi: 10.1177/0899764014558934

Jones, A. C., & Gosling, S. D. (2005). Temperament and personality in dogs (canis familiaris): A review and evaluation of past research. *Applied Animal Behavioral Science, 95,* 1–53.

Lee, T. (2017). Criminalizing fake service dogs: Helping or hurting legitimate handlers? *Animal Law, 23,* 325–354.

Lefebre, S. L., Reid-Smith, R., Boerlin, P., & Weese, J. L. (2008). Evaluation of the risks of shedding salmonellae and other potential pathogens by therapy dogs fed raw diets in Ontario and Alberta. *Zoonoses and Public Health, 55,* 470–480. doi: 10.111/j.1863-2378.2008.01145.x.

Linder, D. E., Siebens, H. C., Mueller, M., Gibbs, D. M., & Freeman, L. M. (2017). Animal-assisted interventions: A national survey of health and safety policies in hospitals, eldercare facilities, and therapy animal organizations. *American Journal of Infection Control, 45,* 883–887. doi: 10.1016/j.ajic.2017.04.287.

Paws & Hearts Animal Assisted Therapy (2019). *Become a volunteer.* Retrieved from www.pawsandhearts.org/volunteer.html

United States Department of Labor, Bureau of Labor Statistics (2013). *Volunteering in the United States – 2013.* Retrieved from https://www.bls.gov/news.release/archives/volun_02252014.pdf

4   Safeguarding the Welfare of Clients and Therapy Dogs

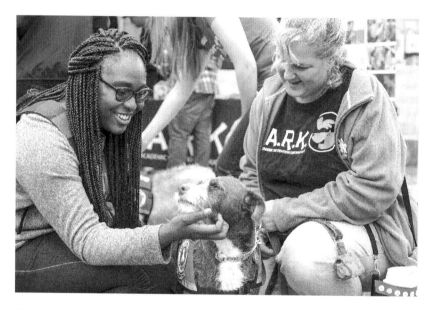

Figure 4.1 Volunteer handler Shelby and her dog, Xena, interact with a student at the University of British Columbia.

Scenario

Billy, a 4-year-old Labradoodle, is an experienced therapy dog and his handler, having had a previous dog credentialed through a well-known, national CAI organization, is experienced as well. Billy participates each week in a program at a seniors' retirement facility and is popular among the residents, many of whom say his visit is the highlight of their week. In fact, they boast about the "Billy Fan Club" they started, complete with photos of Billy and various residents posted at his visitation station within the facility. At Christmas and on Billy's birthday, Billy's handler is overwhelmed by the generosity of the residents who bring gifts for Billy to sessions. As sessions can be busy with multiple residents visiting Billy at the same time, Billy's handler can be distracted by residents' questions and conversations. She recently noticed residents blowing on Billy's face to get him to give them kisses. Reflecting on her life before coming to the retirement home, one elderly resident shared, "This is just what my Yorkie Teddy used to do. It brings me right back to my kitchen and our morning greetings. You know, he was with me for 16 years and I still think about him." Knowing her organization's policy on facial licks, Billy's handler wonders how to curb this behavior without dampening the excitement of Billy's admirers.

Questions for Reflection and Discussion

1. Might therapy dogs learn unintended and unwanted behaviors through their participation in CAIs?
2. How might a handler redirect client behavior that goes against the policy of a CAI organization?

The Burgeoning Field of CAIs

There is little doubt that the field of CAIs has seen a surge in popularity. Though quantifying the number of these programs and the growth of programs over time hasn't been systematically done, there are a few reports in the literature that inform our understanding of just how popular and prevalent CAI programs are, especially in North America. In 2015 Crossman and Kazdin identified over 925 canine visitation programs on college campuses. Haggerty and Mueller (2017) surveyed 150 postsecondary institutions regarding on-campus animal-visitation programs and though the response rate for this study was low, their findings indicate that 62% of the colleges contacted offer some iteration of an animal-visitation stress-reduction program. A web search of CAI organizations revealed but three (curated but nonexhaustive) lists of programs: (1) a list generated by the Animals & Society Institute (2019) that identifies both animal-assisted therapy organizations and training programs; (2) the American Kennel Club (2019), who maintains a list of both national and regional CAI organizations; and (3) a list of animal-assisted therapy (AAT) and reading programs across the United States maintained by an independent organization (Land of Pure Gold, 2019). A recent report on therapy dogs by *National Geographic* (2018) claims there are over 50,000 therapy dogs working in the United States alone. Despite the lack of a comprehensive registry to track CAI organizations, it is safe to say that across community and campus contexts, there has been a proliferation of interest in, and development of, CAI organizations and programs.

Ever-Expanding Contexts for CAIs

As the interest in CAI has grown, so, too, have the contexts within which we find therapy dogs participating in initiatives to boost the well-being of varied community members. Recall the breadth of contexts in which we see CAI teams working in the table we presented in Chapter 1. Though therapy dogs are still popular in elder care facilities to support the well-being of senior citizens, perhaps the best known venue that brings therapy dogs together with clients, therapy dogs can now be found in funeral homes to support mourners, in correctional facilities to support the rehabilitation of inmates, in dentists' offices to support anxious patients, in elementary schools to support reluctant readers, and at the site of tragic events where therapy dogs provide comfort to both people involved in the event and the surrounding community who have come to mourn.

A lot is asked of the CAI teams across these varied contexts. It is especially important to recognize that, across many of these contexts, providing access to therapy dogs is done to support psychosocially vulnerable clients. That is, therapy dogs are brought into these contexts with the specific goal of improving well-being. Thus, in addition to navigating the novelty of the respective setting within which a CAI team must work, there is the added complexity of providing support to clients who are seeking to feel better through their interactions with therapy dogs.

Therapy Dogs in Research

In addition to the varied community settings mentioned previously, we also see CAI teams working to advance the science in support of CAIs as part of research protocols. As the popularity of CAI organizations has grown and the contexts within which we see these programs operate have expanded, there has been a corresponding increase in research done on the effects of CAIs on the well-being of human participants. We now see evidence across contexts and across participants attesting to the benefits of spending time with therapy dogs. As a brief illustration of this, let's look at the titles of recent publications exploring the effects of canines on human well-being.

- "Turning the Page for Spot: The Potential of Therapy Dogs to Support Reading Motivation Among Young Children" (Rousseau & Tardif-Williams, in press).
- "Canine-Assisted Therapy for Children with ADHD: Preliminary Findings From the Positive Assertive Cooperative Kids Study" (Schuck, Emmerson, Fine, and Lakes, 2015)
- "Stepping Out of the Shadows of Alzheimer's Disease: A Phenomenological Hermeneutic Study of Older People With Alzheimer's Disease Caring for a Therapy Dog" (Swall, Ebbeskog, Lundh Hagelin, & Fagerberg, 2017).
- "Petting Away Pre-Exam Stress: The Effect of Therapy Dog Sessions on Student Well-Being" (Ward-Griffin et al., 2018)

What these titles reflect is the range of settings and the variability in clients that therapy dogs find themselves working in and supporting. To safeguard the well-being of therapy dogs, researchers overseeing studies in which therapy dogs are a part are obliged to first apply for research ethics approval through institutional review boards and, second, to report that ethics approval was obtained in subsequent publications of their research. It merits noting that ethics approval helps ensure that therapy dogs working in research initiatives are not put in harm's way and, as part of the application process, asks research-ers to identify protocols they'll implement to safeguard canine well-being dur-ing research activities. As Serpell and colleagues argued in 2010, "Indeed, the use of animals for animal assisted activities and therapy imposes a unique set of stresses and strains on them that the 'industry' is only just beginning to acknowledge" (Serpell, Coppinger, Fine, & Peralta, 2010, p. 497).

Factors Impacting Canine Welfare

As the range of contexts and clients described in the previous sections illus-trate, we see a number of factors that hold the potential to impact the welfare of therapy dogs working in community-based programming, in canine-assisted counseling, or in protocols for scientific research. First, there appears to be ample variability in the training and educational formation of people running and over-seeing CAI organizations. This range includes community volunteers with no formal training in HAIs to highly qualified individuals with PhDs or doctors of veterinary medicine. Just what training should be required to ensure that the protocols followed in screening and selecting therapy dogs and crafting programs for the public are in the best interest of the dogs themselves, the handlers, and the public? A particular challenge in running a CAI organization is that the indi-vidual overseeing the placement of CAI teams in community settings must have expertise in therapy dogs, HAIs, and various dimensions of human well-being.

Second, many CAI organizations can face challenges in finding a space or location to run their CAI programs, keeping in mind that the space must be easily cleaned, accommodate the anticipated number of clients, and not intrude on the day-to-day operations of employees working within the building. As a result, some CAI programs are held in public spaces or commonly shared areas where there is high foot traffic or are integrated into settings with diverse peo-ple, equipment, and sounds. Thus, dogs may be working in spaces where there is little control of external stimuli (e.g., the passing of a noisy janitorial cart, food). Regardless of where therapy dogs might find themselves working, as Serpell and colleagues (2010, p. 483) noted, "Animals need to have an opportunity to habituate to the environment and to the activities in which they are involved."

Third, programs may be intentionally held in public spaces to increase the visibility of the program and to facilitate access to the dogs. One ramification of holding CAI sessions in public spaces is that hazards can be present in the form of dropped medication, food, and office supplies, such as staples, among other hazards. Thus, a key step in safeguarding canine safety is that prior to the arrival of dogs to a venue, the space must be swept or vacuumed to ensure that all hazards have been removed. Related to this, the handler's monitoring of dogs working in public spaces is key to ensuring dog safety and all dogs should have a strong "leave it" response (i.e., a high compliance to this cue) in the event the team encounters a dangerous object or substance when working.

A fourth challenge to canine welfare lies in the profile of the clients that organizations serve. CAI programs are largely implemented to improve the well-being of clients. This is especially true of on-campus canine and airport programs whose aim is to reduce the stress of clients. In these contexts, we see clients with heightened stress interacting with therapy dogs in a public setting. We know that, when stressed, human behavior changes, and we might see, for example, student visitors to a campus canine program engage in stress-influenced behavior (e.g., impatient, highly emotional, agitated). This has implications for the handler, who would need to monitor interactions closely and watch for overly vigorous petting (e.g., roughhousing) or behavior that is out of alignment with program expectations.

The aforementioned challenges and complexities related to therapy dog welfare perhaps raise more questions than answers or guidelines. What is clear is the need for both the careful screening, training, and assessment of CAI teams and the ongoing monitoring of canine well-being to ensure that participation in programming is enjoyable for the dog and presents no threat to dog safety and welfare.

But Does the Dog Want to Do This Work?

Certainly, a key consideration in the field of CAIs is promoting animal welfare. One initial determining question for handlers to consider is whether or not the dog wants to do this work. That is, *Does the dog want to volunteer?* That may seem like a strange question, but it's important to consider. If your dog enjoys being around you and your family but doesn't enjoy meeting strangers, then volunteering with your dog in a public setting to support a variety

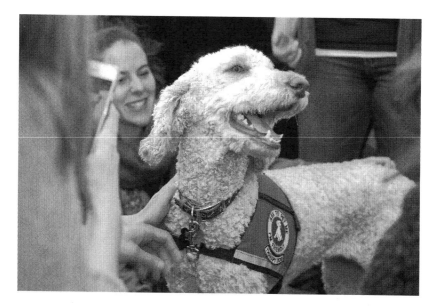

Figure 4.2 Therapy dog Zoe enjoying a session.

of strangers isn't likely going to work. If, however, your dog enjoys meeting strangers and going places outside your home, volunteering may be a good fit for you and your dog. Of course, promoting animal welfare is much more than deciding if your dog would enjoy volunteer work, but it's a starting point. When handlers understand the importance of promoting animal welfare, they will be better equipped to advocate for their dog throughout the screening, training, and assessment processes and within working sessions with clients.

The Importance of Canine Stress Awareness

Research in the area of stress awareness has taken hold within the context of veterinary clinics, and though an emerging area of study, recent work by Scalia and colleagues (2017) investigates the topic of "low-stress handling techniques" or "fear-free principles" as they relate to identifying the preventative measures humans can take in their interactions with dogs to reduce the stress that dogs experience. Other work by Yin (2009) and Overall (2013) advocate more broadly for low-stress handling techniques within clinical settings to avoid animals becoming anxious and associating the clinic with high levels of stress. In the end, an animal characterized by elevated stress presents unique challenges for the clinician seeking to assess health and determine treatment to optimize health. As this relates to therapy dogs, dogs who exhibit low stress are better positioned to provide support to clients, to be engaged with clients, and to respond to handler cues.

With respect to stress education within CAI organizations, a proactive approach is best—that is, standards and policies should be in place a priori to ensure that dogs are being trained and working in conditions conducive to encouraging optimal interactions. Serpell and colleagues (2010, p. 488) paint a rather bleak picture of handlers in their statement: "Unfortunately, many handlers appear oblivious to the stress signals emitted by their animals, perhaps because they enjoy the social aspects of visitation more than their dogs do." What this observation does identify is that handlers must concomitantly monitor their dog's well-being, all the while cultivating and maintaining connections with clients—no small feat! As a starting point, stress education information should be included in the new handler orientation training session so as to equip handlers with information surrounding how to identify indicators of canine stress and how to prevent canines from experiencing elevated stress.

Researchers Iannuzzi and Rowan (1991) were early pioneers in raising awareness around the welfare of therapy dogs working to support client well-being. Their manuscript titled "Ethical Issues in Animal-Assisted Programs" was a first step in bringing animal welfare concerns to the forefront for researchers and practitioners alike. The subsequent echoing of this concern has been repeatedly raised by researchers such as Hatch (2007), Glenk and colleagues (2013, 2014, 2017), and Evans and Gray (2012).

Across publications addressing therapy dog welfare is the issue of canine stress (for a recent review see Silas, Binfet, & Ford, 2019). An overview of the indicators of canine stress is in order. Indicators of canine stress include but are not limited to low body posture, vocalization, turning away, yawning, auto-grooming, pacing, panting, and excessive licking (Beerda, Schilder, van Hooff, de Vries, & Mol, 1998; Rooney, Gaines, & Bradshaw, 2007; Schilder & van der Borg, 2004). Below we offer some of the common ways that therapy dogs might show stress within sessions and the corresponding action that handlers might take to ensure their safety and welfare (see Table 4.1).

Table 4.1 Canine Stress Signals

Stress Signal	Description
PANTING	Dogs pant for natural reasons, such as panting after rigorous playing or when they are hot. Some dogs also pant when they are stressed. If a handler notices that their therapy dog is panting when they are not tired or hot, it's likely that the dog is stressed and needs to take a break from the environment.
TURNING AWAY	Dogs may indicate that they are stressed or do not want to be near a person by turning or moving away from the person. If a handler notices that their therapy dog is turning or moving away, then giving the dog, or encouraging the client to give the dog, an opportunity to move away and come back when the dog chooses is the best option.
PAWING	A dog may place a paw on a person to get the person's attention. This could indicate that the dog is stressed and needs a break or that the dog wants something. A handler can decide if the dog needs a break or wants something and respond accordingly.
WHIMPERING	Sometimes dogs choose to vocalize through whimpering or whining to get a person's attention and indicate that they want something different. This could be due to stress or due to a need (e.g., hunger, wanting a treat). When a dog uses her or his voice to communicate, a handler should consider if he or she needs to respond to stress or to a need (e.g., the dog needs a break) or ignore (e.g., the dog wants your sandwich).
TREMBLING	Typically, dogs don't shake unless they are very cold. Dogs may shake when they are nervous or stressed, though. This is similar to a human's reaction when they are nervous. When a dog is trembling, the handler should remove the dog from the situation immediately.
YAWNING	Dogs hold tension in their jaws. Dogs may yawn to reduce the tension in their jaws. If the handler sees their therapy dog yawn, the handler might consider what was going on and if there was anything or anyone in the dog's environment that could be causing the dog stress.
PACING	When dogs are stressed or overwhelmed, they may pace back and forth. This could be an indication that the dog would like to leave the environment or needs a bathroom break. When a dog is pacing, the handler should offer their dog a break first and then see if the pacing behavior stops.

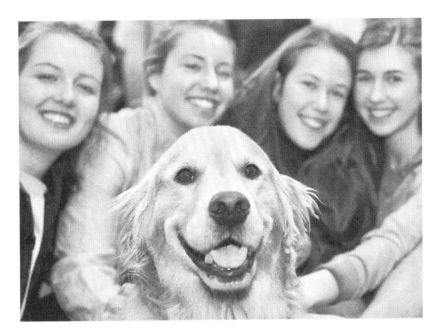

Figure 4.3 Therapy dog Dash smiling.

Of the various indicators of canine stress, it is perhaps lip licking that should be accorded utmost importance. As Scalia and colleagues (2017, p. 22) write, "Lip licking has been previously related to salivary cortisol concentrations in hospitalized dogs (Heckman et al., 2012) and could be useful for the evaluation of acute stress levels in a social context (Beerda et al., 1998)."

Positive Canine Signals

Our focus thus far has been on the importance of recognizing signs of stress in therapy dogs, but handlers should also be on the lookout for signs that dogs are enjoying their interactions with clients—signs that indicate the dog is relaxed, that the dog is interested in seeking interactions with clients, and that the dog is settled in a session. Signs that a therapy dog is settled within a session might include an open mouth, with tongue out, ears forward, and a gently wagging tail, leaning toward the client in a relaxed posture, and demonstrating a play bow.

Do Therapy Dogs Experience Stress in Sessions?

A recent publication by McCullough and colleagues (2018a) explored stress in therapy dogs and garnered press from the likes of *Psychology Today* (2018) and

National Geographic (2018). This latter coverage had a curious title: "Therapy Dogs Work Miracles. But Do They Like Their Jobs?" Using both biomarker (i.e., salivary cortisol) and behavioral indicators of stress in 26 therapy dogs working with pediatric oncology patients in varied health care settings, these researchers concluded, "As hypothesized, results indicate that therapy dogs show minimal signs of distress during AAI sessions, regardless of hospital site" (McCullough et al., 2018a, p. 93). This finding is in accord with previous research, albeit studies that used less comprehensive designs than the design of the McCullough et al. study, all attesting to therapy dogs generally experiencing low stress from participation in canine-assisted programming (e.g., Glenk et al., 2013, 2014; Ng et al., 2015; and Palestrini et al., 2017).

Digging further into the topic of therapy dogs and stress during sessions, it is important to acknowledge that the experimental conditions in which therapy dogs are found to be characterized by low stress may differ markedly from the conditions in which we see therapy dogs participate in community programming. Studies reporting that therapy dogs do not experience stress during sessions are based on scientific investigations in which, we hope, optimal canine welfare practices were implemented (i.e., screened, selected, and experienced CAI teams were used, research ethics applications were submitted, canine stress was monitored during sessions, etc.). As we have argued thus far in this book, there is variability in the training and background of individuals overseeing CAI organizations; variability in the screening, selection, and training of CAI teams; variability in the monitoring of teams working in the field; and diversity in the clients supported by working therapy dogs. Thus, the conditions for studies on therapy dog stress and the day-to-day conditions in which CAI teams work in community programs can and very like do vary considerably. We argue here that there is ample potential for therapy dogs working in community programs to experience stress. Let's look next at possible sources of stress for working therapy dogs.

Potential Sources of Canine Stress

Factors Contributing to Canine Stress

A variety of factors can influence and impact the likelihood that therapy dogs may experience elevated stress. This can include and is not limited to (1) the setting, including the dog's familiarity with the setting and the busyness and noisiness of the setting (e.g., a hospital room versus an airport); (2) how crowded the working conditions are within this setting; (3) the prior experience of the dog and the CAI team; (4) the number of dogs concurrently working in a session and the proximity of dogs to one another; (5) the client profile, including the age of the clients (i.e., young children) and their comfort level and experience with dogs; (6) the number of clients supported within a session; and (7) the duration of the session, as well as the number of sessions in a day.

Handlers as a Source of Therapy Dog Stress?

In recent work out of the University of Milan, researchers Pirrone and colleagues (2017) examined the notion of "social synchrony" within the context of CAI dyads. Social synchrony, or the "coordination of nonverbal behaviors between interactive partners" (Pirrone et al., 2017, p. 45), is akin to *emotional state matching* (Huber, Barber, Farago, Muller, & Huber, 2017) and might help us understand how handlers can transmit positive or negative emotional states to their dogs. Other researchers refer to this as "emotional contagion," in which an individual with elevated stress, for example, can pass stress to others in their immediate environment (Yong & Ruffman, 2014). By videotaping four CAI teams and assessing stress before, during, and after an AAT session through cortisol sampling of dogs and handlers, Pirrone and colleagues explored levels of stress between dogs and handlers during working sessions. Overall, low stress was found in working CAI teams; however, the authors acknowledge

> Dogs are sensitive to their handlers' emotional states (Muller, Schmitt, Barber, & Huber, 2015), and emotional contagion between owners and handlers is possible (Yong & Ruffman, 2014) contributing to the level of emotional disturbance experienced. Thus, dogs may mirror the anxiety and negative expectations of handlers in their cortisol levels, and this could actually happen in the context of AAA, as therapeutic work affects handler-dog teams who work in animal- assisted health care service both emotionally and physiologically (Haubenhofer & Kirchengast, 2007).
>
> (Pirrone et al., 2017, p. 51)

These findings indicate that handlers must be aware and able to respond to their dog's stress, as well as be mindful of their own stress.

Strategies to Mitigate Canine Stress During Sessions

There are a number of steps that CAI organizations and handlers themselves can take to reduce factors that contribute to augmenting the stress of therapy dogs. In a recent publication by Howie (2015), a "Therapy Dog's Bill of Rights" was proffered and included a number of considerations that warrant showcasing here. Howie's recommendations provide guidelines for handlers to consider as a means of gauging their dog's interest in doing therapy work and around ensuring the dog's welfare during working sessions. Key elements in this bill of rights include (1) taking into consideration the dog's perception of the setting ("What might it be like for my dog to walk into this building or room?"); (2) providing assistance to the dog to adapt to the environment ("What might my dog need to become settled in this space?"); (3) focusing on the dog throughout the interaction at least as much as the focus afforded clients and staff; and (4) taking steps to proactively reduce the dog's stress.

Policies that can help mitigate canine stress include

- ensuring that handlers are thoroughly screened and well trained—that they have been selected and prepared for the work they are asked to undertake;
- monitoring the overall number of clients to sessions and the ratio of CAI teams to clients;
- predetermining the duration of the visit so that therapy dogs are not overworked;
- delineating the working session for the dog with a clear beginning (e.g., the placement of the dog's therapy vest) and end (e.g., removal of the vest and possible reward);
- having a program director or organization personnel trained in canine stress indicators monitor dogs for signs of stress;
- ensuring that handlers are trained in the recognition and interpretation of canine stress and behavioral indicators; and
- posting visual reminders of canine stress indicators in the space where programs are held so that individuals participating in sessions are aware of canine stress indicators.

The Importance of Training Handlers in Interpreting Canine Behavior

As part of the training offered to prospective handlers, a CAI organization should ensure that handlers receive information on interpreting canine behavior above and beyond basic indicators of stress. Signs that a dog is disinterested in working or needs a break may include: (1) a change in the dog's baseline or typical behavior; (2) disinterest in greeting a new client; (3) retreating from a client and possibly seeking refuge behind the handler; (4) leaving the area to avoid direct contact or choosing to be away from the client to the extent the leash allows; and (5) having low energy and choosing not to participate in the HAI.

It is important to recognize that when the monitoring of canine stress and behavior is left solely to handlers, handlers might be reluctant to admit that their dog is stressed, as this may be perceived as a sign of incompetence (Ng, Albright, Fine, & Peralta, 2015). Thus, interpreting canine behavior is an important component of handler training as it increases awareness around the well-being of dogs working in sessions and distributes the responsibility of recognizing indicators of canine welfare among all stakeholders.

How Long Should Therapy Dogs Work in a Session?

Just how long should therapy dogs work in any given session? There are a number of factors that influence this decision, including the experience of the CAI team, the context in which the dog is working, the client the dog is supporting, the number of clients supported over the course of a session, and the supervision of canine welfare by CAI organization personnel. As a general rule, the more public the space and the higher the turnover of clients, the shorter the working session for dogs should be. Busy, public settings such as an on-campus library to support college student stress or in an elementary school where the energy of children may run high would be settings where therapy dogs should work shorter sessions. To meet the demand to spend time with therapy dogs and to prevent overtaxing dogs, CAI organization personnel can schedule two shifts with a group of CAI teams arriving halfway through the session to replace teams who began the session.

In addition to the aforementioned factors influencing the decision around how long therapy dogs should work, we can also glean information from published guidelines and from research protocols. In the recently updated white paper by the International Association of Human-Animal Interaction Organizations (IAHAIO, 2018), the following welfare protocol is offered (p. 9):

> Professionals who are responsible for the well-being of the animal during intervention must ensure that the animal is healthy, well rested, comfortable and cared for during and after the sessions (e.g., provision of fresh water, work floors that are safe and suitable). Animals must not be overworked or overwhelmed and sessions should be time limited (30–45 minutes).

It merits noting that this recommended protocol of 30 to 45 minutes per session is for *all* therapy animals working in AAIs and not uniquely or specifically for therapy dogs. Other published guidelines for the duration of sessions can be found in a chapter by Ng and colleagues (2015), who recommend visits of 1 hour with the caveat that this is a rough guideline and factors such as the type of session, number of clients, and activities performed must be taken into account. It also warrants mentioning here that, in some programs, the CAI team participates in multiple, back-to-back sessions on the same day. These may be shorter sessions as are typical of canine reading programs that see a CAI team work in individual sessions with several different children. In this case, the number of sessions must be considered, as well as the total duration a CAI team is asked to work. Monitoring canine well-being when dogs are working in multiple sessions is especially important, as is the tracking of the number of sessions in any given day and throughout the week to avoid overworking CAI teams.

As addressed earlier in this chapter, we have seen an increase in research assessing the effects of CAIs, and we can glean information regarding the duration of sessions from best practices used in peer-reviewed published research. In a randomized controlled trial, Binfet (2017) reviewed the duration of sessions used by researchers who employed, as part of their interventions, therapy dog protocols. As can be seen in Table 4.2, there was ample variation in the length and number of sessions in which therapy dogs were asked to work.

Table 4.2 Summary of Duration and Length of CAIs

Study	Dose Intervention (min)	Number of Sessions per Week	Duration of Intervention (Weeks)	Number of Participants
Variations in dose intervention in randomized controlled trials employing canine-assisted therapy.				
Barker et al. (2015)	10	1	1	40
Barker et al. (2016)	15	1	1	57
Binfet & Passmore (2016)	45	1	8	44
Chu et al. (2009)	50	1	8	30
Crossman & Kazdin (2015)	7 to 10	1	1	67
Fung & Leung (2014)	20	3	7	10
Grajfoner et al. (2016)	20	1	1	132
Havener et al. (2001)	—	1	1	40
Johnson et al. (2008)	15	3	4	30
Martin & Farnum (2002)	15	3	15	10
Schuck et al. (2015)	120 to 150	2	12	24
Vagnoli et al. (2015)	—	1	1	50
Villalta-Gil et al. (2009)	45	2	25	21

Note: Dashes indicate data not reported.

The range of sessions in this body of research varied from 7 minutes to 150 minutes, and determining a conservative duration by averaging the length of sessions reveals a session duration of 33 minutes.

Throughout this book we've made reference to, and provided examples from, the B.A.R.K. program at the University of British Columbia, a program founded and overseen by Dr. Binfet. The weekly drop-in session offered in B.A.R.K. on Fridays and the sessions offered at the local police precinct to reduce officer stress run for 90 minutes. Keeping in mind that optimal welfare conditions are in place for the therapy dogs working in these programs (e.g., CAI teams are carefully selected and trained and have ample prior experience, personnel is on-site to monitor canine stress, etc.), over the 7 years of operation, we have found this duration to work well. Newly accepted dogs who are completing an internship in B.A.R.K. begin with short sessions of 20-minute visits to the lab and work their way up to the 90-minute session over time.

Though longer sessions in research are currently being used (i.e., Ward et al., 2018) who used 90-minute sessions and Pirrone et al., 2017, who used 55-minute sessions that included a 10-minute midpoint break), there has been a recent trend in CAI research to use abbreviated sessions. Palestrini and colleagues (2017) noted that sessions were restricted to 20 minutes for therapy dogs supporting pediatric surgical patients. Other recent work by McCullough and colleagues (2018b) used 20-minute sessions with pediatric oncology patients. Within the context of on-campus stress-reduction programs, we also see abbreviated sessions offered with researchers such as Binfet (2017) using 20-minute sessions, Crossman and Kazdin (2015) using sessions of 7–10 minutes, and Barker, Barker, McCain, and Schubert (2016) using sessions lasting 15 minutes.

As can be seen from the aforementioned review, there is significant variation in the duration of sessions in which therapy dogs find themselves working. Our recommendation is that the duration of a session is determined after careful consideration of the experience of the dog, the busyness of the setting, the number of clients within a session per dog, and the profile of clients seeking support. For a well-screened CAI team working in a setting where canine welfare is monitored by organization personnel and best practice protocols are in place (i.e., termination of the session is possible), sessions of 45–90 minutes are reasonable.

How Many Clients Can a CAI Team Support?

Scanning the relevant literature, there is little published information on the number of clients a CAI team can or should support in a single session. Just as several factors must be considered when determining the duration of a session for working therapy dogs, so, too, must these factors be taken into account when determining the total number of clients a single team should support in a session. High-energy clients such as children or sessions that take place in busy settings (e.g., airports) are key factors reducing the number of total clients with whom a dog should interact. An additional factor adding complexity to the identification of a number of clients is that clients engage with therapy dogs differently—some are happy to have ambient proximity with little or no direct touching whereas other clients can be very tactile and hands-on. Overly interactive clients plus high client turnover must be considered in determining the total number of clients per session. Our recommendation is that handlers carefully monitor therapy dogs for signs of stress during all sessions and that the duration of the session be restricted before dogs become overwhelmed by the number of clients within a session.

Monitoring Canine Well-Being During Sessions

Historically, the focus of CAI organizations has been on ensuring that dogs are well screened and suited to the work they're asked to do. That is, the focus has been on the assessment of dogs *before* they are sent out to interact with the public. Our recommendation is that once CAI teams have been credentialed and assigned to a placement, they are routinely monitored *during* working sessions so that optimal standards of canine welfare can be safeguarded. Dogs may be monitored for indications of stress, handlers might be reminded to toilet or water their dog during longer sessions, and sessions may very well be terminated for CAI teams who are having an off day.

Session Termination Policy

Once signs of stress in a working canine are acknowledged, it is important for procedures and policies to be in place so handlers can act in the best interest of their dog. All CAI organizations should have a session termination procedure. The termination of a CAI session can be externally determined (e.g., when the behavior of the participants makes the visit unsafe or impossible) or internally determined by the handler (e.g., when the therapy dog's behavior suggests he or she is reluctant to work). The following model can be used to determine when to terminate a visit:

- Step 1: Recognize stress indicator(s).

  - Recognize that the dog is unsettled and poorly equipped or positioned to provide support to visiting clients.

- Step 2: Localize the source of canine stress.

  - Is the source external (e.g., the behavior of visiting client) or internal to the dog/handler team?
  - Could the handler's level of stress be influencing canine stress? It is best to have the handler self-regulate stress before the session.

- Step 3: Take the dog out for a break to get away from the source of stress.
- Step 4: Return and reevaluate.
- Step 5: Terminate the session if it is in the best interest of the dog.

  - If the dog is unable to settle, it is best to terminate the session and try again another day.
  - The handler and program coordinator should notice patterns in the dog's behavior over time.

Safeguarding Client or Visitor Well-Being During Sessions

Our discussion thus far has focused on the steps we might take to ensure that the welfare of therapy dogs is monitored and that therapy dogs are working in conditions conducive to their well-being. A related topic worth discussing is the well-being of clients or visitors to CAI programs. Recognizing that CAIs operate to boost the well-being of clients, it is important that client well-being be considered as part of the overall delivery model of CAIs. Certainly, within the context of on-campus programs whose aim is to reduce stress, volunteer handlers are likely to encounter students who may feel hopeless, isolated, and have low overall affect. It could be argued, too, that this client profile could easily be found in the elderly residents of a retirement facility.

We propose a two-pronged approach to safeguarding client well-being during CAI sessions: (1) set behavioral expectations for clients that include guidelines for interacting with dogs and protocols around maintaining hygiene and (2) ensure handlers are sufficiently trained for the context and client population.

Setting Behavioral Expectations for Clients

Certainly, one overlooked aspect of many CAI organizations is the lack of instruction given to clients wishing to interact with dogs. As alluded to previously, we recommend that clients be given instructions on how to interact with dogs within a session and how to maintain optimal hygiene when multiple therapy dogs are working in one setting and a client may visit several dogs. To ensure that clients are prepared for a successful interaction, handlers should, first, teach the client how to greet the dog. This helps establish rapport between the handler and the client and avoids the dog being startled by an overly enthusiastic or excited client. Second, handlers should set parameters for the interaction so clients know to avoid picking up dogs, giving cues to dogs, or feeding dogs (unless instructed), and encourage best practice protocols around hygiene by encouraging clients to disinfect their hands between dog visits.

The education or training of clients described previously around how best to interact with therapy dogs is most effectively done by the handler. This is especially important in stress-reduction programs where clients arriving to canine stations can arrive with elevated levels of stress. This elevated stress can, in turn, alter clients' behavior, and handlers might see increased impatience, frustration, or withdrawal from clients. Setting behavioral expectations for clients may also be important should clients have little prior experience with dogs or have a misguided understanding of how to interact with dogs. As an illustration of this, some international students visiting an on-campus stress-reduction program might have limited hands-on experience with dogs and think that patting (i.e., tapping) a dog's head is how one pets a dog. An experienced handler would redirect the student, demonstrating for the student how to pet the dog by moving the student's hand from the head to toward the tail. This is where the handler's social and emotional skills are brought into action and a handler might use directive yet supportive language to encourage appropriate client-dog interactions (e.g., "Oh, let me show you how to pet Billy in a way he really enjoys.").

Our opening scenario in which Billy, the Labradoodle working in a seniors' retirement facility, was being conditioned to lick the faces of clients is another illustration of an opportunity for the handler to educate clients in appropriate client-dog interaction. Redirecting client enthusiasm to engage with dogs is a key component of a hander's responsibility. In response to clients who blow on a dog's face to elicit a kiss, a handler might say, "Let's not blow on Billy's face as he'll learn to kiss anyone who brings their face near him. Instead, why don't I show you how he likes to greet new people."

Can Clients Teach Therapy Dogs Bad Habits?

An unexplored aspect of the therapy dog's experience is the possibility that dogs will learn bad habits through their interactions with the public. The previous illustration of clients blowing on a dog's face to elicit a kiss is but one example of this and though no account of therapy dogs learning bad habits from their work with clients could be identified in the anthrozoological or veterinary behavioral literature, handlers might see therapy dogs learn any number of undesired behaviors. This might include any of the following: (1) facial licks in response to clients blowing on the dog's face, (2) clients muddling a dog's response to a handler's cues by using inconsistent verbal and hand cues to have dogs perform tricks, (3) clients introducing and teaching the dog new (possibly undesired) tricks, (4) dogs seeking and accepting food from strangers in programs where the administration of dog treats is allowed, and (5) a constant seeking of touch or the inability to remain calm without constant physical reassurance with the therapy dog repeatedly pawing for attention.

The Importance of Handler Training

The most effective way of ensuring that client welfare is safeguarded is to ensure that handlers are well trained to support the clients within the context the CAI team is working. This would include educating handlers around the rationale for bringing dogs to the setting, the need for support (i.e., what dimension of well-being needs boosting?), and any potential characteristics or particularities that characterize the client (e.g., children with autism may make random vocalizations and the CAI team is not to be startled or surprised by this).

As an illustration of this, the Building Academic Retention Through K9s (B.A.R.K.) program at the University of British Columbia referenced previously and mentioned in the previous chapter, invites its more than 60 handlers to participate in a variety of programs—some with young children in the community in a program titled "Building Confidence Through K9s," in which children from an after-school program are bussed to campus to build leadership skills and our regular weekly stress-reduction drop-in program to support university student well-being.

Handlers working in the after-school program required training on setting boundaries for children during their interactions with their dogs. For example, this included teaching the children about how best to pet their dog and establishing a greeting that did not include a hug between the child and the handler as this ran counter to the guidelines of the after-school organization. Sometimes the training for handlers can be incorporated with the training provided to clients. In this program for example, a discussion of how to greet one another could be led with the entire group.

Within our on-campus stress-reduction program, handlers are invited to receive "QPR" training to better understand college student mental health. QPR (question, persuade, refer) follows a format similar to the well-known CPR resuscitation model, however, within the context of suicide prevention. During training, handlers increase their comfort level in talking about self-harm and suicide and are reminded of the importance of identifying clients who appear in distress, alerting B.A.R.K. staff, and redirecting these clients to additional mental health resources. Readers curious to learn more about QPR are directed to the QPR Institute (https://qprinstitute.com/).

Conclusion

All stakeholders, whether they be involved in the selection and screening of CAI teams or involved in overseeing the delivery of CAIs to support client well-being, bear a responsibility to ensure that the welfare of therapy dogs remains a top priority. Certainly, steps can be taken around ensuring that dogs who are selected to participate in programs are well suited to the work they are asked to do; however, measures can be taken once dogs are credentialed and working to ensure that dogs do not experience elevated stress during sessions and are working in conditions that allow them to optimally support the well-being of clients.

References

American Kennel Club (2019). *AKC recognized therapy dog organizations*. Retrieved from www.akc.org/sports/title-recognition-program/therapy-dog-program/therapy-dog-organizations

Animals & Society Institute (2019). *Animal-assisted therapy programs*. Retrieved from www.animalsandsociety.org/human-animal-studies/animal-assisted-therapy-programs

Barker, S. B., Barker, R. T., McCain, N. L., & Schubert, C. M. (2016). A randomized cross-over exploratory study of the effect of visiting therapy dogs on college student stress before final exams. *Anthrozoos, 29,* 35–46. doi: 10.1080/08927936.2015.1069988.

Barker, S. B., Knisely, J. S., Schubert, C. M., Green, J. D., & Ameringer, S. (2015). The effect of animal-assisted intervention on anxiety and pain in hospitalized children. *Anthrozoos, 28,* 101–112.

Beerda, B., Schilder, M. B., van Hooff, J. A. R. A. M., de Vries, H. W., & Mol, J. A. (1998). Behavioural, saliva cortisol and heart rate responses to different types of stimuli in dogs. *Applied Animal Behaviour Science, 58,* 365–381.

Binfet, J. T. (2017). The effects of group-administered canine therapy on university students' wellbeing: A randomized controlled trial. *Anthrozoos, 30,* 397–414. doi: 10.1080/08927936.2017.1335097.

Binfet, J. T., & Passmore, H. A. (2016). Hounds and homesickness: The effects of an animal-assisted therapeutic intervention for first-year university students. *Anthrozoos, 29,* 441–454.

Chu, C. I., Liu, C. Y., Sun, C. T., & Lin, J. (2009). The effect of animal-assisted activity on inpatients with schizophrenia. *Journal of Psychosocial Nursing and Mental Health Service, 47*(12), 42–48. doi: 10.3928/02793695-20091103-96.

Crossman, M., & Kazdin, A. E. (2015). Animal visitation programs in colleges and universities: An efficient model for reducing student stress. In A. H. Fine (Ed.), *Handbook on animal-assisted therapy: Foundations and guidelines for animal-assisted interventions* (pp. 333–337). New York: Elsevier.

Evans, N., & Gray, C. (2012). The practice and ethics of animal-assisted-therapy with children and young people: Is it enough that we don't eat our co-workers? *British Journal of Social Work, 42,* 600–617.

Fung, S., & Leung, A. S. (2014). Pilot study investigating the role of therapy dogs in facilitating social interaction among children with autism. *Journal of Contemporary Psychotherapy, 44,* 253–262. doi: 10.1007/s10879-014-9274-z.

Glenk, L. M. (2017). Current perspectives on therapy dog welfare in animal-assisted interventions. *Animals, 7,* 7–24. doi: 10.3390/ani7020007.

Glenk, L. M., Kothgassner, O. D., Stetina, B. U., Palme, R., Kepplinger, B., & Baran, H. (2013). Therapy dogs' salivary cortisol levels vary during animal-assisted intervention. *Animal Welfare, 22,* 369–378.

Glenk, L. M., Kothgassner, O. D., Stetina, B. U., Palme, R., Kepplinger, B., & Baran, H. (2014). Salivary cortisol and behavior in therapy dogs during animal-assisted interventions: A pilot study. *Journal of Veterinary Behavior, 9,* 98–106.

Grajfoner, D., Harte, E., Potter, L., & McGuigan, N. (2016). The effect of dog assisted intervention on wellbeing, mood and anxiety. *International Journal of Environmental Research and Public Health, 13*(1), 1–6. Retrieved from: http://www.mdpi.com/jounral/ijerph

Haggerty, J. M., & Mueller, M. K. (2017). Animal-assisted stress reduction programs in higher education. *Innovations in Higher Education, 42,* 379–389. doi: 10.1007/s10755-017-92930-0.

Hatch, A. (2007). The view from all fours: A look at an animal-assisted activity program from the animals' perspective. *Anthrozoos, 20,* 37–50.

Havener, L., Gentes, L., Thaler, B., Megel, M. E., Baun, M. M., Driscoll, F. A., . . . Agrawl, N. (2001). The effects of a companion animal on distress in children undergoing dental procedures. *Comprehensive Pediatric Nursing, 24,* 137–152. doi: 10.1080/01460860118472.

Heckman, J. P., Zaras, A. Z., & Dreschel, N. A. (2012). Salivary cortisol concentrations and behavior in a population of healthy dogs hospitalized for elective procedures. *Applied Animal Behavior Science, 141,* 149–157.

Howie, A. R. (2015). *Teaming with your therapy dog.* West Lafayette, Indiana: Purdue University Press.

Huber, A., Barber, A. L. A., Farago, T., Muller, C. A., & Huber, L. (2017). Investigating emotional contagion in dogs (*Canis familiaris*) to emotional sounds of humans and conspecifics. *Animal Contagion, 20,* 703–715.

Iannuzzi, D., & Rowan, A. N. (1991). Ethical issues in animal-assisted therapy programs. *Antrhozoos, 4,* 154–163. doi: 10.2752/089279391787057116.

Johnson, R., Meadows, R., Haubner, J., & Sevedge, K. (2008). Animal-assisted activity among patients with cancer: Effects on mood, fatigue, self-perceived health, and sense of coherence. *Oncology Nursing Forum, 35,* 225–232. doi: 10.1188/08. ONF.225-232.

Kirchengast, S., & Haubenhofer, D. K. (2007). Dog handlers and dogs' emotional and cortisol secretion responses associated with animal-assisted therapy sessions. *Society and Animals, 15,* 127–150. doi: 10.1163/156853007X187090.

Land of Pure Gold (2019). *Assisted-Animal Therapy & R.E.A.D. (Reading Education Assistance Dogs) Group Listing.* Retrieved from http://landofpuregold.com/rxb.htm

Martin, F., & Farnum, J. (2002). Animal-assisted therapy for children with pervasive developmental disorders. *Western Journal of Nursing Research, 24,* 657–670. doi: 10.1177/019394502320555403.

McCullough, A., Jenkins, M. A., Ruehrdanz, A., Gilmer, M. J. Olson, J. . . . O'Haire, M. E. (2018a). Physiological and behavioral effects of animal-assisted interventions on therapy dogs in pediatric oncology settings. *Applied Animal Behavior Science, 200,* 86–95. doi: 10.16/j.applanim.2017.11.014.

McCullough, A., Ruehrdanz, A., Jenkins, M. A., Gilmer, M. J., Olson, J. . . . O'Haire, M. E. (2018b). Measuring the effects of an animal-assisted intervention for pediatric oncology patients and their parents: A multisite randomized controlled trial. *Journal of Pediatric Oncology Nursing, 35,* 159–177. doi: 10.1177/1043454217748586.

Muller, C. A., Schmitt, K., Barber, A. L., & Huber, L. (2015). Dogs can discriminate emotional expressions of human faces. *Current Biology, 25,* 601–605. doi: 10.1016/j.cub.2014.12.055.

National Geographic (2018, May 1). Therapy dogs work miracles. But do they like their jobs? Retrieved from https://news.nationalgeographic.com/2018/04/animals-dogs-therapy-health-pets/

Ng, Z., Albright, J., Fine, A. H., & Peralta, J. (2015). Our ethical and moral responsibility: Ensuring the welfare of therapy animals. In A. Fine (Ed.), *Handbook on animal-assisted therapy: Foundations and guidelines for animal-assisted interventions* (4th ed., pp. 357–376). Burlington, MA: Academic Press. http://dx.doi.org/10.1016/B978-0-12-801292-5.00026-2.

Overall, K. L. (2013, September 1). *Fear factor: Is routine veterinary care contributing to lifelong patient anxiety?* Retrieved from http://veterinarynews.dvm360.com/fear-factor-routine-veterinary-care-contributing-lifelong-patient-anxiety

Palestrini, C., Calcaterra, V., Cannas, S., Talamonti, Z., Papotti, F., Buttram, D., & Pelizzo, G. (2017). Stress level evaluation in a dog during animal-assisted therapy in pediatric surgery. *Journal of Veterinary Behavior, 17,* 44–49. doi: 10.1016/j.jveb.2016.09.003.

Pirrone, F., Ripamonti, A., Garoni, E. C., Stradiotti, S., & Albertini, M. (2017). Measuring social synchrony and stress in the handler-dog dyad during animal-assisted activities: A pilot study. *Journal of Veterinary Behavior, 21,* 45–52. doi: 10.1016/j.jveb.2017.07.004.

Psychology Today (2018, January 3). *Do therapy dogs suffer from stress when they are working?* Retrieved from www.psychologytoday.com/us/blog/canine-corner/201801/do-therapy-dogs-suffer-stress-when-they-are-working

Rooney, N. J., Gaines, S. A., & Bradshaw, J. W. S. (2007). Behavioural and glucocorticoid responses in dogs (Canis familiaris) to kenneling: Investigating mitigation of stress by prior habituation. *Physiology & Behavior, 92,* 847–854.

Rousseau, C. X., & Tardif-Williams, C. Y. (in press). Turning the page for Spot: The potential of therapy dogs to support reading motivation among young children. *Anthrozoos.* Early online edition.

Scalia, B., Alberghina, D., & Panzera, M. (2017). Influence of low stress handling during clinical visit on physiological and behavioural indicators in adult dogs: A preliminary study. *Pet Behaviour Science, 4,* 20–22. doi: 10-.21071/pbs.v0i4.10131.

Schilder, M. B. H., & van der Borg, J. A. M. (2004). Training dogs with help of the shock collar: Short and long term behavioural effects. *Applied Animal Behaviour Science, 85,* 319–334. doi: 10.1016/j.applanim.2003.10.004.

Schuck, S. E. B., Emmerson, N. A., Fine, A. H., & Lakes, K. D. (2015). Canine-assisted therapy for children with ADHD: Preliminary findings from the Positive Assertive Cooperative Kids Study. *Journal of Attention Disorders, 19,* 125–137. doi: 10.1177/10870547113502080.

Serpell, J. A., Coppinger, R., Fine, A. H., & Peralta, J. M. (2010). Welfare considerations in therapy and assistance animals. In A. Fine (Ed.), *Handbook on animal-assisted* therapy: Theoretical foundations and guidelines for practice (pp. 481–503). New York: Elsevier.

Silas, H. J., Binfet, J. T., & Ford, A. (2019). Therapeutic for áll? Observational assessments of therapy canine stress in an on-campus stress reduction program. *Journal of Veterinary Behavior: Clinical Applications and Research, 32,* 6–13. doi: 10.1016/j.jveb.2019.03.009

Swall, A., Ebbeskog, B., Lundh Hagelin, C., & Fagerberg, I. (2017). Stepping out of the shadows of Alzheimer's disease: A phenomenological hermeneutic study of older people with Alzheimer disease caring for a therapy dog. *International Journal of Qualitative Studies on Health and Well-Being, 12,* 1347013. doi: 10.1080/17482631.2017.1347013.

Vagnoli, L., Caprilli, S., Vernucci, C., Zagni, S., Mugnai, F., & Messeri, A. (2015). Can presence of a dog reduce pain and distress in children during venipuncture? *Pain Management Nursing, 16,* 89–95. doi: 10.1016/j.pmn.2014.04.004.

Villalta-Gil, V., Roca, M., Gonzalez, N., Domenec, E., Cuca, E., Escanilla, A., . . . Sch-Can group. (2009). Dog-assisted therapy in the treatment of chronic schizophrenia inpatients. *Anthrozoos, 22,* 149–159. doi: 10.2752/175303709X434176.

Ward-Griffin, E., Klaiber, P., Collins, H. K., Owens, R. L., Coren, S., & Chen, F. S. (2018). Petting away pre-exam stress: The effect of therapy dog sessions on student well-being. *Stress and Health, 34,* 468–473. doi: 10.1002/smi.2804.

Yin, S. (2009). *Low stress handling, restraint and behavior modification of dogs and cats: Techniques for patients who love their visits.* Davis, CA: Cattle Dog Publishing.

Yong, M. H., & Ruffman, T. (2014). Emotional contagion: Dogs and humans show a similar physiological response to human infant crying. *Behavioural Processes, 108,* 155–165. doi: 10.1016/j.beproc.2014.10.006.

5 Best Practices in Canine-Assisted Intervention Team Training

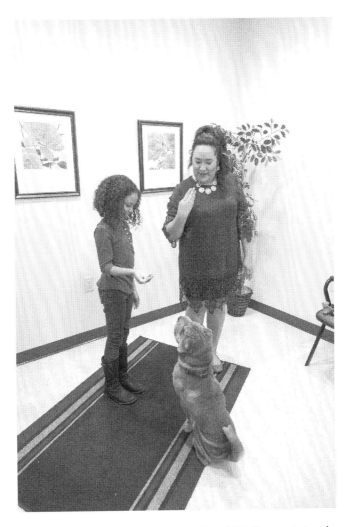

Figure 5.1 CAC practitioner Sarah Moreno and a child client training therapy dog Zeus.

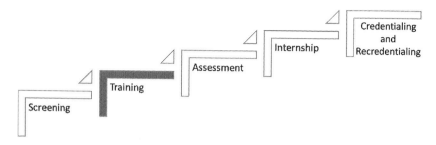

Figure 5.2 CAI team credentialing process.

The field of CAIs is flourishing with organizations providing support to a range of clients in a variety of settings. In response to this surge in popularity, there is a need to explore how both handlers and therapy dogs can be trained for CAI work. The aim of this chapter is to present best practices in CAI team training as a means of preparing teams for assessment. We will review the key components in training CAI teams and, in doing so, will lay a foundation for Chapter 6 that explores training for CAC teams in mental health settings.

Scenario

Carol and her standard poodle sailed through the dog obedience classes offered at her local community center. Her dog, Fred, seemed to love learning and picking up new skills. Eager to extend her work with Fred, Carol underwent training to become a volunteer CAI handler with a local organization in her city. On the day of the assessment, when Carol was asked to demonstrate a series of skills with Fred, it was clear that Fred was the best-behaved dog in the batch of prospective therapy dogs being assessed that day. Fred, always with his eyes on Carol, awaiting his next cue, wasn't fazed by any of the tasks he was asked to do. At the end of the session and to Carol's complete surprise, Carol was told by the director of the CAI organization that she and Fred were not a match for the work they do, as Fred had little interest in interacting with anyone other than Carol. Carol knew he was attached to her but wondered if she'd trained Fred's interest in others out of him by having him repeatedly focus on her as she taught him one skill after another.

Questions for Reflection and Discussion

1. How important is obedience training for CAI teams?
2. What skills should handlers and therapy dogs learn and practice that support strong CAI work?
3. How might handlers and dogs be trained to encourage interactions with strangers?

How Much Training Is Needed?

There is great variability in both the amount and type of training provided by CAI organizations. In our research on published requirements for CAI organizations, we found that 47% of programs offered no training to prospective CAI teams (Hartwig & Binfet, 2019). Our findings also revealed variations in CAI training, including no training, brief online training, one-day training, or comprehensive CAI team training. Considering that CAIs require handlers to work with a different species (i.e., canines) and there are complexities that arise when humans work alongside animals, we believe that CAI organizations should provide comprehensive training to potential teams. Comprehensive training involves training the potential handler and therapy dog over the course of multiple sessions, depending on a team's skill level and training needs, so that teams can develop competencies for CAI work.

Components of Effective Team Training

We propose that effective training for CAI teams involves three components: (1) knowledge, (2) skills, and (3) practice (see Figure 5.3). Next, we review each of these within the context of preparing prospective CAI teams for their assessment leading to becoming a credentialed CAI team:

- **Knowledge**: CAI handlers need to understand the foundations of CAIs, information about the organization for whom they are volunteering or around the CAI practice they would like to use in their professional work, and knowledge about working with and training dogs.
- **Skills**: CAI teams (the handler and the dog) need to learn the skills they will use in CAI work and for which they will be assessed. We argue for transparency here on the part of the CAI organization so that prospective CAI teams are not surprised by the assessment process.
- **Practice**: CAI teams need opportunities to practice skills prior to being assessed and working with clients in real-world settings. These three components are, of course, important on their own, but it is important to recognize that they are also mutually informing.

As an illustration of the interplay among the three dimensions of training, consider that the more a handler knows about canine stress signals, the more the handler can learn to interpret canine behavior and then can practice skills for responding to canine stress within the context of client interactions. CAI organizations should strive to develop knowledge, skills, and opportunities to practice skills for all CAI teams prior to assessing teams.

In addition to addressing these three components of CAI team training, we posit that the more specialized the CAI practice, the more that CAI handlers need to be trained on honing their specialized skills to support client well-being. Comprehensive team training allows CAI organization trainers

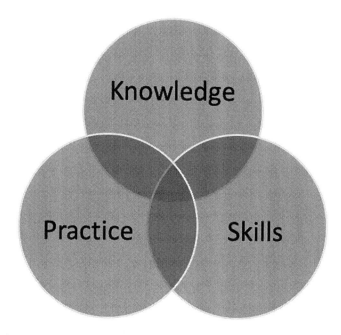

Figure 5.3 Components of effective training.

and evaluators to track each team's progress, target specific areas of growth, identify teams that are a poor fit for therapy work, and continually monitor the skills and dispositions of potential teams as they make their way toward being assessed for credentialing. We now examine each of these components of the training process in depth.

Knowledge: Training the Handler

This section will focus on knowledge content areas that are important for handlers to master as part of the training process. These include CAI organization training and understanding the philosophy of dog training methods.

CAI Organization Training

CAI organizations should provide handlers with foundational training in CAIs, written guidelines explaining policies and procedures, expectations for handlers, and helpful information that sets teams up for success in their CAI work. Pet Partners, a large U.S. animal therapy organization, provides a handler guide that covers a myriad of topics related to the services they provide. The handler guide includes information about the Pet Partners mission and goals, handler responsibilities, suitability and health requirements for animals, team assessment information and scoring, best practices for facility visits, considerations for successes and challenges in facilities, and resources needed (Pet Partners, 2017). Their guide provides handlers with detailed information and examples, so that the handlers know what to expect in the team assessment and facility visits. As many local CAI organizations operate on shoestring budgets and with limited resources, we recognize that the information provided to handlers will vary. Nevertheless, we recommend that CAI organizations address the following topics with prospective CAI teams in training:

- **Program basics:** Every organization has their own story about how they were established and the type of services they offer. As handlers are ambassadors for organizations, it's important for handlers to know the organization's mission or vision statement, policies, and procedures. CAI organization trainings should cover mission and goals, overview of programs offered, staff member roles and contact information, and client demographic information.
- **Handler job description:** Handlers should understand their responsibilities with their dog, their responsibilities as handlers within the CAI organization, and as a volunteer or practitioner working with clients. It's important for handlers to be aware of and embrace CAI organization rules and policies that clarify expectations such as dress code, cell phone use, photography policies, gift giving, and food/drink policies.
- **Therapy dog job description:** As discussed in Chapter 3, dogs need certain skills and temperament for CAI work. In this section, CAI organizations can provide guidelines for what skills and temperament attributes therapy dogs need to have to work with specific clients served by the organization.
- **Facility or practice logistics:** CAI teams work in a variety of facilities and practice settings. It's helpful for the CAI organization to provide specifics about facility expectations, schedules, important dates, arrival and departure procedures, volunteer coordinator contact information including an emergency contact number, and client challenges and needs.
- **Safety/incident report procedures:** Prevention is key, but sometimes safety concerns or ethical issues can arise, even with the most well-trained teams. CAI teams should be prepared to handle ethical issues; procedures for mandated reporting of abuse or neglect; what to do if a client, dog, or staff member is hurt; and how to promote safety at all times.
- **Success stories:** CAI organizations benefit when stories of the successful work of their CAI teams are shared. The purpose of this section is to share with handlers the options they have around sharing positive interactions and achievements in working with clients, policies around how the program obtains client permission for sharing photos and stories, and policies governing handlers' use of social media.

When CAI organizations take the time to teach potential teams about their mission, goals, policies, and procedures, CAI teams can be optimally prepared to follow procedures and equipped to handle challenging situations once out in the field.

Philosophy of Humane Training Practices

In the HAI and canine behavior literature, there has been a surge of research on humane training practices for dogs in general (e.g., British Columbia Society for the Protection of Animals, 2018) and more specifically for therapy dogs (e.g., Howie, 2015). Humane training practices are important for CAI organizations and potential teams because CAI handlers should use evidence-informed, nonaversive, and humane practices to train their dogs as they prepare for assessments leading to becoming a credentialed CAI team. In the 1960s, Pryor (2002) transformed the field of animal training through her work with dolphins using force-free operant conditioning. In her book, she introduced a positive reinforcement training concept called "clicker training," in which trainers use a clicker to provide an auditory reinforcement for the desired behavior, which is then followed by a reward, such as a treat. A key point in her book is that trainers should focus on what the animal is to learn and reinforce that behavior rather than punishing an animal for not complying. Pryor proposed that clicker training can teach a dog, at any age, to learn a variety of skills and behaviors. Another animal behaviorist, Patricia McConnell (2002), explored the differences between humans and dogs and how much can be learned from understanding the dogs, especially around their behaviors and communication.

In her book *The Other End of the Leash*, McConnell (2002) guides dog owners in learning what they can do on the human end of the leash to have a positive relationship with their dogs. As handlers explore training philosophies and options to hone their and their dog's skills in preparation for CAI assessment, we encourage handlers to ask themselves, What kind of relationship do I want with my dog? If handlers want a relationship with their dog built on positive interactions and trust, then they should use training methods grounded in positive, trust-enhancing methods.

Skills: Preparing for CAI Training

Socialization

The first step in training a dog begins with proper socialization. Puppies experience three crucial periods of social development: the primary, socialization, and enrichment periods (Howell, King, & Bennett, 2015). The primary period lasts from birth to 3 weeks of age. During this period, the puppy is primarily dependent on their mother. The socialization period occurs from 3 to 12 weeks of age, and sometimes up to 14 weeks of age. The enrichment period lasts until a dog reaches sexual maturity. Although all of these periods of development are important, the socialization period is a critical time for puppies. According to Howell and colleagues (2015), the socialization period begins with puppies interacting and learning from their littermates. At approximately 5 weeks of age, puppies begin to be fearful of new and unfamiliar environments and noises (Scott & Fuller, 1965). This fear response can become permanent and puppies can struggle to develop attachments with humans and potentially develop behavioral problems if they do not have exposure to humans before 14 weeks of age when the socialization period ends (Freedman, King, & Elliot, 1961; Serpell, 2016). Researchers have found that puppies who are handled by humans and gently exposed to new sounds and experiences are able to be less fearful in new environments and more affiliative with humans (Battaglia, 2009; Gazzano, Mariti, Notari, Sighieri, & McBride, 2008).

For prospective handlers interested in partnering with their dog for CAI work, socialization has important implications in preparing therapy dogs to withstand the stressors and stimuli they will encounter. If handlers have the opportunity to adopt a dog as a puppy, they can try to ensure that the puppy receives optimal socialization, either from the breeder or adoption facility and then subsequently within the context of the handler's own home. Regardless of whether the handler obtains her or his puppy from a breeder or a rescue facility, the handler should gather as much information about the puppy's socialization prior to bringing the puppy home.

One socialization program that some breeders use is called Puppy Culture (2017). This program offers videos, books, and other resources to support puppy socialization. Breeders who use this program gently handle the puppies, use recordings to expose the puppies to new sounds, and spend time playing with the puppies. When puppies are brought home, owners can continue socialization by playing their puppy, introducing the puppy to new people, housetraining outside using lots of treats, and replacing chewing behaviors with acceptable toys. All of these socialization activities help puppies connect with their owners and learn from an early age how to be behaviorally successful in their homes.

If handlers have adopted an older dog, they still have an opportunity to support the dog's socialization. Dog behaviorists, such as Karen Pryor (2002) and the late Sophia Yin (2011), encourage dog owners to go slowly in introducing their dog to new environments and to work on small behaviors first. Working with a private trainer to assess the dog for temperament and behavior may be a good first step prior to introducing the dog to unfamiliar people and places. Although we know that dogs can be wonderful companions, a therapy dog requires specialized skills and dispositions. Dogs who demonstrate aggressive behaviors or excessive fear are not a good fit for CAI work. In our respective programs, when we assess teams and see prospective dogs display problematic behavior, we share with handlers that some dogs are a better fit as a family pet and are may not be suited to working as part of a CAI team.

Preparing for CAI Team Training

Training Supplies

There are several items handlers need in order to train their dog for CAI work. We recommend handlers support their dog's training by having the following close at hand:

- water and water bowl (dogs should always have access to water before and after training)
- treats (low value, such as kibble, to high value, such as pieces of ham or chicken)
- clicker (if applicable)
- waste bags
- brush (for on-the-spot grooming, if needed)
- hand sanitizer
- towel (to clean paws, as needed)
- wet wipes (optional; these can be helpful for wiping hands, slobber, or dirty surfaces)

Handlers are encouraged to create a "training kit" so these supplies can be easily transported.

Dog Attire

In addition to the aforementioned items, both members of the CAI team should be appropriately dressed. Dogs should be equipped with the following:

- standard nylon or leather collar (no choke, prong, or e-collars), harness, or gentle leader
- 4- or 6-foot leash (no retractable leashes; the dog needs to be near the handler and dogs must be able to practice skills while leashed)
- a training bandana or vest (optional; some handlers use a training bandana or vest as a way to let the dog know they are "going to work, which this can be helpful in setting up a routine for training and eventually for therapy work)

Human Attire

Handlers will want to wear clothes that allow them to move freely, get on the ground if needed, and get dirty, as dog training can sometimes be a messy process. Clothing considerations for handlers include the following:

- comfortable and flexible pants (e.g., jeans, leggings, sweatpants, or slacks)
- T-shirt, polo shirt, or a shirt that can get dirty (shirts can get wet or dirty in training from wet dog noses, mouths, and paws)

- close-toed shoes (e.g., tennis shoes, flats, loafers; handlers should wear shoes that provide stability, that allow handlers to move quickly, e.g., if handlers must quickly remove a dog from a situation, and that protect toes from paws and dropped items)

Handler attire should be comfortable and flexible and offer support.

Choosing a Trainer

In this section we're going to discuss how handlers can choose a trainer and how organizations can provide a trainer that will best prepare handlers and dogs for the CAI team and future CAI work. As we noted at the outset of this chapter, the training provided to prospective CAI teams varies. When training is offered, some CAI organizations only provide training for the handler and expect that the potential handler will be responsible for the training of the dog (either alone or with assistance from a trainer). Certainly, one aim of this chapter is to encourage transparency on the part of CAI organizations around their training and assessment expectations for prospective CAI teams.

CAI organizations can best prepare potential CAI teams by providing training to both the human *and* canine partners. This allows the organization to control the training methods encouraged between handlers and dogs (i.e., positive reinforcement and fear-free training methods) and helps ensure that the organization's trainers are well qualified to work with potential teams. We recognize that some CAI organizations may not have the capacity to provide training to both handlers and dogs. However, if the goal is to train prospective CAI teams for successful work as a credentialed CAI team working on behalf of a CAI organization, putting best practices in place would see that both the hander and the dog receive training. For potential teams who are looking to volunteer with CAI organizations who do not offer training for both the human and the canine partners, teams should seek out positive reinforcement and fear-free dog trainers who may help them with their mastery of the foundational obedience training needed for successful CAI work.

Handlers seeking to work with a trainer to prepare for a CAI assessment might consider a trainer who is a certified pet dog trainer (CPDT). This certification is earned through the Certification Council for Professional Dog Trainers (CCPDT). CPDT candidates have to demonstrate their training abilities through an examination, 300 hours of dog training experience, and a signed attestation from a CCPDT certificant and agree to uphold the CCPDT Standards of Practice and least intrusive, minimally aversive (LIMA) Policy (CCPDT, 2014). It bears mentioning that not all CPDTs use positive reinforcement–only methods. We recommend that handlers interview several trainers before choosing one. To discern trainer compatibility, handlers can ask questions such as "How would you describe your training approach?" "Do you use positive reinforcement methods?" and "Do you use choke, prong, or e-collars in your training?"

Prerequisite: Basic Obedience Skills

One approach that we recommend for CAI organizations is to employ a basic obedience test as a prerequisite for teams interested in becoming CAI credentialed. This allows prospective teams to demonstrate basic obedience skills prior to working on CAI skills. By using basic obedience as a prerequisite, CAI organizations have some level of assurance that teams who do not have basic skills and may not be a good fit for therapy work do not begin the process of CAI team training. The basic obedience evaluation that we recommend to screen potential teams is the Canine Good Citizen (CGC) test, which was developed by the American Kennel Club (AKC) in 1989. The CGC test was originally used as a tool that would support family dogs in having good manners in the home and community (AKC, 2018a). In a national survey of animal-assisted interaction (AAI) organizations, Linder, Siebens, Mueller, Gibbs, and Freeman (2017) identified that 33% of AAI organizations required only a CGC certificate for their CAI teams, even though the CGC certificate was not originally intended to assess suitability for CAI-related work. We do not recommend that CAI organizations use only the CGC test as an indicator or measure of CAI team suitability. To be clear, we recommend that CAI organizations use the CGC test as a prerequisite prior to beginning CAI team training.

The CGC test is composed of 10 skills. We'll describe these skills in the context of the CGC test, just as if an evaluator were facilitating the test. The CGC skills (AKC, 2018b) include the following:

1. Accepting a friendly stranger: The evaluator walks toward the team and greets the handler by shaking hands and exchanging verbal greetings. The dog should stay calmly next to the handler and show no signs of fear, aggression, or shyness.
2. Sitting politely for petting: The dog sits calmly next to the handler while the evaluator pets the dog. The dog does not retreat from the evaluator and shows no signs of fear, aggression, or shyness.
3. Appearance and grooming: The dog appears healthy and groomed and does not react or retreat when being brushed or touched by the evaluator.
4. Out for a walk: The dog walks on a loose leash next to the handler. The team follows the evaluator's directions to do a right, left, and about turn as well as one stop, during which the dog stops when the handler stops.
5. Walking through a crowd: The dog walks on a loose leash next to the handler in a crowd, passing at least three people who walk in front of, or behind, the team.
6. Sit and down on cue and staying in place: The dog's leash is replaced with a 20-foot leash. The dog sits on cue, then moves to a down on cue. Then the dog stays in a sit or down on cue while the handler walks 20 feet away from the dog, holding onto the long leash, and then returns to the dog.

7. Come when called: The handler gives a stay cue, walks 10 feet away from the dog, turns to face the dog, and cues the dog to come.
8. Reaction to another dog: The team approaches another team with a neutral dog. The handlers shake hands and exchange pleasantries, then continue walking past each other for 10 feet. The dog should have no or a minimal reaction to the neutral dog and the other handler.
9. Reaction to distractions: The evaluator presents visual (e.g., a person walks in front of the dog) and auditory distractions (e.g., a person drops a crutch that makes a loud noise). The dog may show interest or be slightly startled but should not try to run away or react with aggressive behavior.
10. Supervised separation: The dog stays with the evaluator while the handler goes out of sight for three minutes. The dog has no or minimal reaction to the handler being out of sight.

For the CGC test, there are no pretest training requirements for handlers or dogs, and the teams must pass all skills in the assessment in order to receive the CGC certification. The CGC skills are intended to represent skills that well-adjusted dogs should have whether they are at home or in a public setting.

Practice: Developing CAI Team Skills

CAI teams are routinely asked to work with diverse clients in a variety of settings. Preparing teams for this kind of work requires teams be trained beyond what is typically done to ensure dogs are well behaved at home or on a walk in the neighborhood. As we review each of the skills that follow, you'll notice that some of the CAI team skills are similar to the skills required by the CGC test. These skills warrant emphasis in CAI training as it's important that teams can demonstrate skills consistently as they prepare for the CAI assessment. Further, some of the skills we recommend are assessed in different or nuanced ways and thus are distinguished from the assessment used as part of the CGC test.

You will notice that we emphasize practicing these skills in a training setting prior to the CAI team assessment. We believe that the best way to prepare teams for a CAI assessment is to practice skills with a CAI organization trainer who can provide feedback and support, as this person will understand how the skills will be assessed. This allows the trainer to help each prospective CAI team develop, troubleshoot, and hone skills that are needed for CAI work prior to the team assessment. Handlers can use treats, verbal cues, and other positive reinforcement during their practicing of skills. We recommend that once dogs are able to respond correctly to a cue on a consistent basis, handlers can reduce their use of reinforcements. The skills described next are presented for development alongside a trainer. These are the same skills that will be discussed in Chapter 7 for the CAI team assessment.

Skill 1: Handler Check-In

Taking time to verbally check in with the handler and review paperwork is a helpful way to start the assessment, as this can put the handler at ease. It's also a natural way a team might begin a visit, by greeting a volunteer coordinator at a facility and reviewing paperwork. In the assessment, this is an ideal time for the evaluator to assess if the handler is dressed appropriately and the dog is wearing an approved collar and leash. We believe that the *handler check-in* is a valuable skill.

To practice this skill in training, the trainer should welcome the team to a practice space, similar to the room in which the team might be evaluated. During this practice, the handler should be dressed in attire approved for CAI work. The handler should also make sure that the dog is wearing an approved collar and leash. The trainer should verbally greet the handler and review paperwork without approaching the team (that skill follows next). During training, the handler doesn't actually need paperwork, but during the assessment, the handler may be required to bring the canine health screening form, a training certificate of completion, and a completed CAI team information form.

Skill 2: Accepting a Friendly Stranger

One of the most important skills that a therapy dog should have is a willingness to meet and be around strangers. CAI teams typically meet strangers in the environments that they visit, such as hospitals, universities, or airports. Thus, handlers and therapy dogs must be assessed on how they respond when someone they don't know approaches them.

To practice this skill, the dog should be cued to sit or stand next to the handler. Handlers can use treats and cue the dog to stay while practicing this skill. When the team is ready, the trainer can approach the handler, shake the handler's hand, and say hello. The goal of this skill is for the dog to be able to remain next to the handler without approaching, reacting, or jumping on another person who approaches.

Skill 3: Teaching How to Greet a Dog

Whether they are clients, patients, or members of the public, not everyone necessarily knows how to greet a dog. McConnell (2002) described how dogs may demonstrate stress signals when they are pet on the head, hugged, given direct eye contact, or approached from the front. Yin (2011), in her advice on greeting a dog, recommended that people ask to pet the dog first, approach the team slowly from the side, stand still and allow the dog to smell the newcomer, and then pet the dog gently, provided the dog looks relaxed. Both of these dog behaviorists emphasize that dogs should be greeted in the way the dog generally likes to be greeted (i.e., let the dog approach the human) and pet them in places they like to be pet (i.e., gently and not on the head).

To practice this skill, the trainer can approach the team and ask if she or he can pet the dog. The handler can acknowledge that the trainer would like to meet the dog, and tell the trainer that dogs have a certain way they like to be greeted. The handler can then teach the trainer to stand still while the dog sniffs the trainer. While the dog is sniffing the trainer, the handler can tell the trainer that the next step is for the trainer to bend down, let the dog approach, and pet the dog on the chest or the back (or wherever the dog really likes to be pet). The handler can reinforce to the trainer that the dog really enjoys greeting people and being pet in that way.

 ### Skill 4: Sit

Basic obedience skills are some of the most helpful skills for CAI work. We want dogs to demonstrate natural dog behaviors, such as a dog's excitement to meet someone new, yet we also need dogs to be calm and adaptable, especially in potentially busy or chaotic environments.

The purpose of practicing this skill is to get the dog in a sit position for the subsequent skill, which is handling. It's also helpful to practice this skill to make sure that the dog responds consistently to the sit cue because therapy dogs often need to sit during CAI work for a variety of reasons. To practice this skill, the handler will cue the dog to a sit position. The dog should be focused on the handler after the dog moves to a sit position. It might be helpful during practice to rehearse this skill with other distractions, such as people walking past the team. Although the purpose of this skill is not to assess for distractions, there will be times in CAI work where therapy dogs may need to sit with distractions happening around them.

 ### Skill 5: Handler

It's important that CAI teams are assessed for how they respond to the dog being touched and handled by another person. This skill is important because most clients or visitors want to pet therapy dogs and may touch dogs in places that they do and don't want to be touched. Handlers should train their dog to be receptive to touch by the handler and by others. In doing so, the dog will become conditioned to accept petting and touching in different places. Handlers should still direct clients to not touch areas in which the dog does not like to be touched and intervene immediately if a client touches the dog in a place or way that makes the dog uncomfortable.

To practice this skill, the dog will already be in a sit position. The trainer and handler will kneel next to the dog. The handler should have her or his

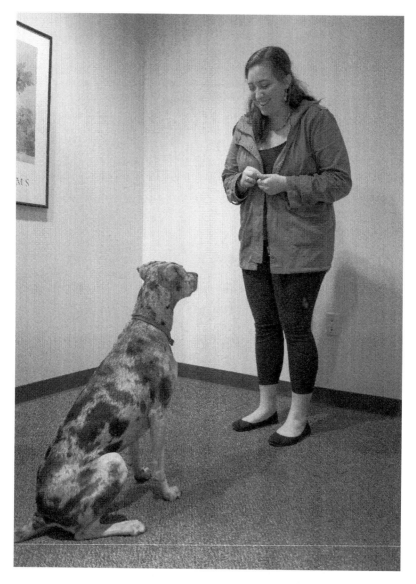

Figure 5.4 Shelby Lowe practicing the sit cue with therapy dog Daemon.

hands on their dog the entire time during this skill. The handler should also talk to both the dog and the trainer during the skill. The trainer will pick up and/or touch each paw; look in the dog's eyes, ears, and mouth; and rub along the dog's back and tail. The handler should assist the trainer by offering to open the dog's mouth or lift the dog's ears.

Skill 6: *Down*

As mentioned previously, basic obedience skills are helpful for busy CAI environments. Teaching a dog to go to a down position can be helpful for allowing others to pet the dog or for having the dog settle while the handler discusses something with a client or facility staff member.

This skill was described in the CGC test. The purpose of reassessing this skill is to get the dog in a down position for the next skill, which is grooming. To practice this skill, the handler will cue the dog to a down position. The dog should be able to stay in a down position for several seconds to begin the next skill.

Skill 7: *Grooming*

For this skill, the team is being assessed to determine whether the dog appears healthy and groomed. An unhealthy or ungroomed dog may be a dog that hasn't had a bath recently, has fleas, or has open wounds. An unhealthy dog can transfer sickness or disease to vulnerable humans (i.e., children and patients in hospitals or nursing homes). This skill also considers how the dog responds to being lightly brushed with a soft-bristle brush.

This skill was briefly described in the CGC test. The purpose of reassessing this skill is to verify that the handler maintains the dog's health and grooming during training and, eventually, during the assessment and future CAI services. The dog should already be in a down position and the handler and trainer can be sitting or kneeling next to the dog. The trainer will brush the dog lightly a few times with a soft-bristle brush. Just like in the handling skill, the handler should talk to the trainer and dog, be in proximity with the dog, and support the trainer and dog interaction during brushing.

Skill 8: Walking on a Loose Leash

During CAI visits, handlers must be able to manage their dog for a variety of reasons. Some people have dog allergies or are afraid of dogs and do not want to be approached by a dog. Sometimes there is equipment, such as medical equipment, that the dog could get tangled in, which could be potentially painful and harmful to the patient. A therapy dog should be able to walk calmly by the handler's side, not pulling or dragging behind, demonstrating to people in the facility that both the handler and dog are walking and working well together and that the handler is in control of the dog's behavior at all times.

This skill was described in the CGC test. Handlers should practice this skill by training their dog to walk next to them. There are several techniques for teaching a dog to walk next to the handler, such as offering the dog treats every few steps or changing directions if the dog starts to walk in front of the handler. During this skill, the leash should be loose between the handler and dog, where the leash drops down and looks like a J-shape between where the handler is holding the leash and where it is attached to the dog. The dog should be able to walk calmly next to the handler when the handler makes turns in different directions and stop when the handler stops. The handler should talk to the dog during this skill and let the dog know when the handler will be getting ready to make turns or stop. This skill demonstrates that the handler and dog are focused on one another and the dog will allow the handler to lead in both relaxed and stressful situations.

 ## Skill 9: Walking Through a Crowd

In CAI work, teams must be prepared for walking in crowds and having several people approach the dog at once. Sometimes teams need to be able to walk through busy halls or places where a lot of people are walking. It's appropriate for handlers to wait until crowds disperse or people walk by, but in both common and emergency situations, a therapy dog should be able to safely walk in a crowd alongside the handler. Assessing for how the handler and the dog manage crowds is imperative. We believe that all CAI programs should evaluate how handlers and dogs walk in crowds and manage several people approaching and wanting to pet the dog.

This skill was briefly described in the CGC test. Once the team has mastered the skill of walking on a loose leash, then practicing walking through a small (three-person) crowd is a good next step. The team should practice by walking in a straight line for 15 to 20 feet while people walk in front of or behind the team. The handler should talk to the dog during this skill to let the dog know that people are walking in front and behind the team but that the team is going to keep walking forward. The dog should be able to stop when the handler stops, if needed, to let someone pass by during this skill.

 ## Skill 10: Managing Several People Who Want to Pet the Dog

One skill used by some CAI organizations is a skill we'll refer to as being *petted by several people*. This skill involves at least three people asking to pet the dog: one person standing, one sitting in a chair or wheelchair, and one sitting or kneeling on the floor. The purpose of this skill is to see how the team responds when people crowd around the dog. We believe that a CAI team skill that is more important than being crowded by people is to assess the handler's ability to manage and set limits when several people want to pet the dog at the same time. The handler has the right to decide how many people can pet the dog at the same time and how they should be positioned. This skill can be assessed by observing how the handler manages a group of people, ideally spacing people out and allowing the dog to approach each person to receive petting. Facilitating the skill in this way shows the handler's ability to be assertive and establish boundaries, prevents the dog from being crowded, and helps safeguard canine welfare.

As many CAI teams end up volunteering in facilities or at events in which children are present (Fredrickson-MacNamara & Butler, 2010), we believe the assessment of this skill is an ideal time to identify how a team responds to a child between the ages of 6 and 12 approaching the team. The child volunteer should be able to be calm and follow the guidance of the evaluator and handler. Also, many CAI settings will see the CAI team interact with diverse members of the public. The team can and should practice this skill with people who are different ages, sexes, ethnicities, abilities/disabilities, and sizes. If the dog is reactive to a certain type of person during practice, such as a man with a beard or hat, then the handler should consult a trainer to assess for reactivity with potential CAI recipients before continuing with training.

To practice this skill, the trainer should have three volunteers who are willing to help with this skill. The trainer can tell the handler that all three people would like to pet the dog. The handler will acknowledge that all three people would like to pet the dog and ask them to spread out next to each other, shoulder-width apart. The people can sit down on the floor, in chairs, or stand. The handler will practice teaching all three people how to greet a dog (as presented in the *teaching how to greet a dog* skill). The handler can then allow the dog to sniff and greet each person. In the assessment, the team should be assessed with three people, one of whom is a child between the ages of 6 and 12, and an individual using a wheelchair. If the team can practice with a person using a wheelchair during training, the handler can bring the dog next to the person in the wheelchair or pick the dog up, if the dog is small enough.

 ## Skill 11: Reaction to Distractions

Distractions are a normal part of life. Our family lives, work settings, and social time are filled with unexpected people and events and can include people coming to our front door, the pinging of text messages, and sudden loud noises. In facilities where CAI teams work, there are many potential distractions, some that are typical and some that are startling, for both handlers and therapy dogs. These distractions may be auditory distractions (e.g., the noise from a dropped item, people screaming or shouting, and loud announcements) and/or visual distractions (e.g., people who sound or move differently, people running, and people using mobility aids including crutches or motorized wheelchairs). The purpose of practicing, and later assessing, how handlers react to distractions is to see if handlers can support their dog during unexpected instances or events. The purpose of exploring how dogs react to distractions is to see if dogs are able to remain calm, have an initial reaction, and recover or if they become aggressive or are unable to recover from the distraction. Some dogs respond to loud noises by eliminating or startling to the point of not recovering. Because loud noises happen, therapy dogs have the right to be surprised but then should be able to continue walking and recover. In this skill, we recommend assessing the team's reaction to distractions that would be commonly found in facilities in which a CAI team might work (e.g., a person hurriedly running by, such as a doctor, nurse, or child getting to another destination, and the sound of a vacuum).

To practice this skill, the handler should talk to the dog and continue walking with the dog. If the dog is startled by either distraction, the handler can pause to redirect the dog's focus, support the dog, and continue walking. It may be helpful for the handler and dog to practice this skill out in public, where there are other distractions, such as walking around a store where there are sounds and people passing by.

 ## Skill 12: Reaction to a Team With a Neutral Dog

Another type of distraction is the presence of other dogs (i.e., service dogs working in the facility, pet dogs, or other therapy dogs). With the popularity of helping dogs in the public increasing, it's important that therapy dogs are assessed for their reaction to a neutral dog. The assessment of this skill is important as it helps engender the safety and welfare of all people and animals within the facility. Therapy dogs need to be predictable in their behavior. This requires therapy dogs to be nonreactive around dogs who themselves may be working. We referred earlier in this chapter to the importance of socialization in puppyhood, and introducing puppies to a variety of other nonaggressive dogs can play a role in shaping a dog's reaction to other dogs later in life.

Related to this, the ideal therapy dog should have a stronger focus on humans (i.e., the handler, clients) than on other dogs in the vicinity. Certainly, a therapy dog cannot have an aggressive reaction to other dogs, but they must also not have a keen interest in other dogs who happen to be nearby. This skill takes practice and can be one skill that clearly indicates if a dog is suitable for CAI work. There are different ways in which this skill can be assessed, such as the CAI team stopping to talk to another team or the CAI team just passing by another team with a neutral dog. This can be done initially with a wide berth between dogs. As our goal is to comprehensively assess CAI teams, we believe that therapy dogs should be able to pass by and be near another team for a brief amount of time without reacting to, or showing a keen desire to interact with, a neutral dog.

To practice this skill, the handler should observe how her or his dog responds around other dogs in a safe and predictable setting. Attending a basic training course with other dogs might be a helpful way to initially evaluate interdog reactivity. When training for this skill, the dog should be focused on the handler. Initial training should involve a dog just being in the presence of another dog, without walking by another team. The training can then progress to walking past another team with a 10-foot distance between the teams. The distance can be reduced over time and with practice but should never be close enough that the dogs could reach each another. If a dog is reactive (i.e., lunging and barking) to other dogs, we encourage handlers to reconsider CAI work. Teams will have achieved competency in this skill when the dog can sit quietly next to the handler while the handler briefly talks to another handler with a dog that is several feet away.

Skill 13: Stay

It's beneficial for a therapy dog to have mastered a reliable *stay* cue. Remaining in a *stay* is important because there are times when the handler may need to talk with someone without the dog walking around or interacting with anyone else. The dog may also need to stay if something spills or drops that the dog should avoid.

This skill was described in the CGC test. To practice this skill, handlers should cue the dog to *sit* and then cue the dog to *stay* without the handler moving. The handler can then cue the dog to *stay* and take one small step backward. The dog should be reinforced each time for staying in a sit position and not getting up. Handlers can gradually increase their distance from their dog and increase the time their dog is asked to hold a *stay* position. In order to be successful in developing a consistent *stay*, it's important that in the beginning handlers build this skill incrementally, starting with only short distances (e.g., 1 to 2 feet) and short durations.

Skill 14: Come When Called

The *come when called* behavior is an important skill should a dog become separated from the handler or the handler needs to call the dog away from a person, food, object, or other animal. The *stay* and *come when called* skills can be assessed one right after the other.

This skill was described in the CGC test. Once dogs have a consistent *stay*, then they can practice the *come when called* skill. The handler will cue the dog to *stay* and then call the dog to *come*. Some trainers recommend that the handler turn and face the opposite direction while looking back, as if the handler is getting ready to run away from the dog. This may invite the dog to think that the handler wants to play chase and motivate the dog to move toward the handler. The handler could also just stand still, facing the dog, and call the dog's name or cue the dog to *come* in a positive or excited tone of voice. The handler should reinforce the dog for coming once the dog has come all the way to the handler to the point where the handler can gently touch the dog's collar.

Skill 15: Setting a Limit – Restraining Hug

CAI teams are responsible for facilitating interactions with a variety of people, many of whom require nuanced interactions to ensure the interaction is safe and that the welfare of the therapy dog and clients is considered. As such, it is important that handlers have skills for setting limits with, and managing requests by, CAI clients. The next two skills allow the handler to demonstrate these skills. One model for setting limits is called the ACT model, developed by Landreth (2012). The model has three steps:

- A: Acknowledge the person's wishes or wants.
- C: Communicate the limit.
- T: Target an alternate behavior.

One example of when we might see the need for a handler to set a limit is when a client wants to touch the dog in a way that the dog doesn't like, such as a restraining hug. Rather than allowing a dog to be hugged in that way, a better option is to set a limit. To redirect the client, the handler might say the following:

- A: "Sandy, I can see that you'd like to hug Harvey."
- C: "But Harvey is not for hugging like that."
- T: "You can pet his back or give him a belly rub. That's how Harvey likes to be pet."

The ACT model is a helpful tool, as needed, for setting limits with CAI clients.

To train for this skill, teams need to practice using the ACT model. Some handlers may feel uncomfortable interrupting a person who is moving to do something with the dog, but it's important for handlers to be able to establish boundaries around the interactions clients have with their dogs. If handlers are working with older CAI clients, such as college students, it's appropriate to change the language to fit better for that population. The handler could say something like, "Harvey really likes getting pet on her back instead of getting a human hug. I know you just want to connect with him, so I'm letting you know what way he likes to be touched."

 ### Skill 16: Setting a Limit – Request to Take Dog

Sometimes handlers are asked to allow things that go against CAI organization policy. Often these requests have good intentions but are not clearly thought out. One example is a volunteer coordinator at a facility asking if she or he can take the dog into a staff-only area to greet the staff. This would be unethical, because it would give the volunteer coordinator the responsibility of handling the dog. This situation also presents a host of hazards, such as the dog experiencing stress or the coordinator or staff being injured by the dog. CAI handlers need to be prepared to respond to requests such as this, and using the ACT model is a helpful way to do this. If a client were to approach a handler and ask if they could take the therapy dog, Harvey, on a walk, the handler could respond in this way using the ACT model:

- A: "I can see that you'd really like to walk Harvey by yourself."
- C: "But Harvey has to stay with me at all times."
- T: "Harvey and I can go on a walk with you within the facility."

This skill can be used for other requests, but this skill is important to teach, have handlers practice, and then assess. It is especially important that handlers be prepared to set limits in different ways because there are a variety of inappropriate ways in which people may want to interact with a therapy dog, jeopardize organization ethics, and/or could cause stress or harm to the dog.

 Skill 17: Leave It

Reinforcers, such as toys and treats, can be beneficial tools to encourage canine play and teach dogs new skills. At facilities, some items may appear to be toys or treats that really are not to be used by dogs in that way. Examples of this include medication or food accidentally dropped on the floor, stuffed animals that belong to child clients, and balls used for physical therapy. It's important for dogs to learn that some items are off limits, and there are also times when it's permissible to interact with these items. The cue *leave it* is often used to teach dogs when to leave an item alone. We believe this skill is important for CAI teams because in facilities there may be many things that can be dropped on the floor or viewed by dogs as something they can sniff, eat, or play with that can be unsafe and even dangerous. Therapy dogs should also learn this skill with food so that if they come across food or medication in a facility, the handler can use this cue.

To practice this skill, handlers should begin by practicing with an object that the dog doesn't particularly like. It could be a paperweight or brick. The handler can practice walking by objects like this and using the *leave it* cue so that the dog becomes used to walking by an object without giving it attention. The handler can slowly replace boring objects with objects that are of increasing interest. This might include toys with which the dog likes to play, followed by food the dog doesn't like (that would be safe to eat), and finally food the dog likes. Another helpful aspect of training for this skill is distance. Handlers can first start by placing an object 15 feet away, then when that is successfully ignored, pass a few feet closer to the object. The handler should eventually be able to pass by an object that the dog likes without the dog responding to the object when the *leave it* cue is given.

 Skill 18: Accepting a Treat

The *leave it* skill teaches a dog to avoid a reinforcer; however, the *accepting a treat* skill assesses how the team manages another person giving the dog a reinforcer. Allowing others to give treats can be beneficial in developing and enhancing a therapy dog's relationship with clients. Many people don't know how to give treats to dogs correctly, so this skill provides the handler with an opportunity to teach a client how to give their dog a treat. We believe this skill is important to assess in teams that may use treats as part of their CAI sessions (i.e., where treats are used to help create a bond between the client and a therapy dog). We agree that this skill should be optional, as some handlers do not want another person giving their dog treats while they are volunteering.

To practice this skill, handlers can teach others how to give a treat to their dog. They can do this by asking the trainer or a volunteer to cue the dog to sit, put the treat in the center of their hand with their fingers together, and then gently lower their hand underneath the dog's mouth. The dog should practice sitting or doing a desired behavior in order to receive the treat.

There are other skills that dogs may need to learn in order to be work effectively in specialized settings. For example, in a hospital, where employees may use a variety of equipment as part of their daily work duties while a team is visiting a client, dogs should be assessed for their reaction to the specialized equipment found in this setting. In Chapter 8 we'll discuss assessment consideration across a variety of specialized contexts.

Conclusion

We've covered a great deal of information in this chapter. We started by exploring the framework of CAI team training: knowledge, skills, and practice. We then examined the knowledge that handlers need to effectively facilitate CAIs, including content that CAI organizations can cover in an orientation. We discussed the philosophy of humane training practice and how positive reinforcement can enhance the handler-canine relationship. We then discussed the importance of socialization and the tools needed to prepare for CAI training. Finally, we provided a description of basic obedience prerequisite skills and CAI teams skills that should be developed and honed for CAI work with diverse clients in varied settings.

This chapter focused solely on training handlers for the CAI team assessment and to work in volunteer settings. Our next chapter looks specifically at training for professional CAI teams working in the mental health field, specifically canine-assisted counseling (CAC) teams.

References

American Kennel Club (AKC). (2018a). *Canine Good Citizen (CGC)*. Retrieved December 30, 2018, from www.akc.org/products-services/training-programs/canine-good-citizen/

American Kennel Club (AKC). (2018b). *CGC test items*. Retrieved December 30, 2018, from www.akc.org/products-services/training-programs/canine-good-citizen/training-testing/

Battaglia, C. L. (2009). Periods of early development and the effects of stimulation and social experiences in the canine. *Journal of Veterinary Behavior: Clinical Applications and Research, 4*(5), 203–210.

British Columbia Society for the Protection of Animals (2018). *Review of dog training methods: Welfare, learning ability, and current standards*. Retrieved from https://spca.bc.ca/wp-content/uploads/dog-training-methods-review.pdf

Certification Council for Professional Dog Trainers (CCPDT). (2014). *Dog trainer certification*. Retrieved January 4, 2019, from www.ccpdt.org/certification/dog-trainer-certification/

Fredrickson-MacNamara, M., & Butler, K. (2010). Animal selection procedures in animal-assisted interaction programs. In A. H. Fine (Ed.), *Handbook on animal-assisted therapy: Theoretical foundations and guidelines for practice* (3rd ed., pp. 111–134). New York: Academic Press.

Freedman, D. G., King, J. A., & Elliot, O. (1961). Critical period in the social development of dogs. *Science, 133*, 1016–1017.

Gazzano, A., Mariti, C., Notari, L., Sighieri, C., & McBride, E. A. (2008). Effects of early gentling and early environment on emotional development of puppies. *Applied Animal Behaviour Science, 110*(3–4), 294–304.

Hartwig, E. K., & Binfet, J. T. (2019). What's important in canine therapy? An investigation of canine-assisted therapy program online screening tools. *Journal of Veterinary Behavior, 29*, 53–60.

Howell, T., King, T., & Bennett, P. (2015). Puppy parties and beyond: The role of early age socialization practices on adult dog behavior. *Veterinary Medicine: Research and Reports, 6*, 143–153. doi: 10.2147/VMRR.S62081.

Howie, A. R. (2015). *Teaming with your therapy dog*. West Lafayette, IN: Purdue University Press.

International Association of Animal Behavior Consultants (IAABC). (2018). *Hierarchy of procedures for humane and effective practice*. Retrieved December 20, 2018, from https://m.iaabc.org/about/position-statements/lima/hierarchy/

Landreth, G. (2012). *Play therapy: The art of the relationship* (3rd ed.). New York: Brunner Routledge.

Linder, D. E., Siebens, H. C., Mueller, M. K., Gibbs, D. M., & Freeman, L. M. (2017). Animal-assisted interventions: A national survey of health and safety policies in hospitals, eldercare facilities, and therapy animal organizations. *AJIC: American Journal of Infection Control, 45*(8), 883–887. doi: 10.1016/j.ajic.2017.04.287.

McConnell, P. B. (2002). *The other end of the leash: Why we do what we do around dogs*. New York: Ballentine Books.

Pet Partners. (2017). *Pet Partners handler guide*. Bellevue, WA: Pet Partners.

Pryor, K. (2002). *Don't shoot the dog!: The new art of teaching and training*. London: Ringpress Books.

Puppy Culture. (2017). *What is Puppy Culture?* Retrieved January 4, 2019, from www.puppyculture.com/

Scott, J. P., & Fuller, J. L. (1965). *Genetics and the social behavior of the dog*. Chicago, IL: University of Chicago Press.

Serpell, J. (2016). *The domestic dog: Its evolution, behavior and interactions with people* (2nd ed.). Cambridge: Cambridge University Press.

Yin, S. A. (2010). *How to behave so your dog behaves*. Neptune City, NJ: T.F.H. Publications.

Yin, S. A. (2011). *How to greet a dog poster*. Retrieved December 22, 2018, from http://info.drsophiayin.com/greeting-poster

6 Canine-Assisted Counseling

Preparing Teams for Clinical Work

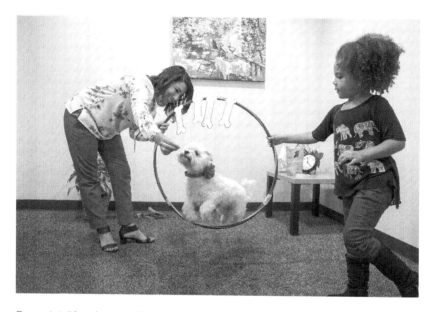

Figure 6.1 Play therapist Celeste Johnson and a child client help therapy dog Vera Wang do the "hula challenge."

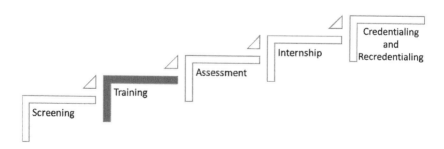

Figure 6.2 CAI team credentialing process.

The aim of this chapter is to delve into the practice of canine-assisted counseling (CAC). The chapter begins by providing a definition of CAC, review literature in this field, and discuss why CAC teams need to develop competence prior to working with clients. We will then present a framework for CAC training that meets ethical standards for developing competence in a specialized field. Finally, we'll present and describe the CAC Skills Checklist, a form that can be used to assess skills for CAC sessions. CAC is a practice in which practitioners are responsible for supporting vulnerable clients working on mental health goals, thus the need for comprehensive training for both practitioners and dogs is essential. This chapter will explore preparing CAC teams for clinical work with clients. Consider the following scenario.

Scenario

Jessica, a 13-year-old, has been struggling with depression for several years. The depression began when her parents divorced 3 years ago. The depression worsened when her grades declined 2 years ago and when, last year, she did not make the basketball team. Jessica's mom asked Jessica if she would be willing to go to counseling with a mental health practitioner who has been trained to provide CAC with a therapy dog named Holly. Jessica tells her mom that she is curious about working with a dog but not sure how she feels about going to a counselor. Jessica decides to try counseling for a few sessions. In the first session, Jessica learns how to greet Holly. Holly is a honey-colored goldendoodle, who wags her tail and appears excited to play with Jessica. As the session begins, Jessica and the counselor sit down on the floor with Holly and do a therapeutic activity in which they all take turns answering questions on a Thumball™, which is similar to a soccer ball with prompts, such as "Favorite Movie." Jessica thinks it's funny that they get to brainstorm how Holly might respond to the Thumball™ prompts. After that activity, the counselor and Jessica discuss what goals Jessica would like to work on and how Holly might be a part of working on those goals. The counselor shares with Jessica that there are a lot of different ways in which Holly can be involved in counseling, such as expressive art and mindfulness activities, to support Jessica in working toward her clinical goal. Holly can also be a support to Jessica by being there to play with and pet while Jessica and the counselor talk about goal-related issues. Jessica decides she would like to come back and work with the counselor and Holly.

Questions for Reflection and Discussion

1. How is having the therapy dog, Holly, helpful to Jessica in the counseling process?
2. What kind of specialized training does the counselor need in order to have Holly present in counseling sessions and meet ethical standards for mental health practitioners?
3. What skills should the counselor be able to employ in sessions to promote the client-canine relationship and prevent harm to the client and therapy dog?

What Is Canine-Assisted Counseling?

CAC is an emerging practice in the field of CAIs. As presented in Chapter 2, CAC is a goal-directed process in which a mental health practitioner and therapy dog work as a team to use the therapeutic powers of human-animal interaction to help clients resolve mental health and behavioral challenges and achieve growth. The practice of CAC encompasses other professional terms, such as canine-assisted psychotherapy, canine-assisted therapy in counseling, animal-assisted counseling (AAC), and canine-assisted play therapy; however, to maintain consistency the term CAC is used throughout this book. Figure 6.3 below provides an overview of where CAC is situated within the broader context of CAIs.

In this book we make a purposeful distinction between canine-assisted therapy (CAT) and CAC because practitioners in each field provide services that meet different client goals and the ways in which the therapy dogs are involved also differs. In reviewing the Pathways to Well-Being model, the goals for CAT are focused on physical or rehabilitation goals, whereas the goals for CAC are focused on mental health goals. In CAT settings, CAI teams trained for volunteer settings often partner with rehabilitation therapists. The work the CAI team does in this context may need to follow structured protocols in order to provide support to clients. For example, a therapy dog and handler may need to walk slowly next to a person who is re-learning how to walk. In this CAT setting, the dog is on a leash and is focused on providing a service that supports a rehabilitation goal. In contrast, in CAC settings, practitioners often work with their own dog, not a separate CAI team. Therapy dogs in CAC settings tend to be more mobile (i.e., off leash), have more choice about how to be involved in CAC interventions, and participate actively with clients based on client goals. By allowing therapy dogs in CAC settings to be mobile and interactive, there is increased risk as issues could arise if therapy dogs are insufficiently trained. For example, a child client struggling with behavioral

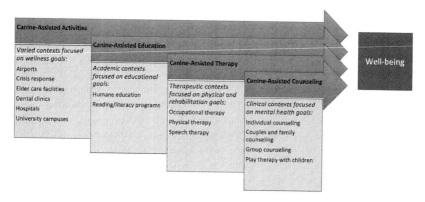

Figure 6.3 Pathways to well-being model.

issues may try to play too roughly with a therapy dog, offer the dog a crayon to eat, or throw a puppet at the therapy dog. In working with clients of any age, clinicians need to prevent and be prepared to set limits on interactions that could be harmful for the client or dog. Thus, in this chapter we aim to provide a comprehensive overview of CAC training and skills that are needed for teams working in mental health settings.

A Review of CAC Literature

One of the first clinical uses of CAC was written by Levinson (1969), who allowed his dog, Jingles, to be present for counseling sessions. In one example, Levinson reports that a mother and child, who had struggled in reaching his clinical goals, showed up several hours early for a session. Levinson writes,

> While I greeted the mother, Jingles ran right to the child and began to lick him. Much to my surprise, the child showed no fright, but instead cuddled up to the dog and began to pet him. When the mother wanted to separate the boy from the dog, I signaled for her to leave them alone.
>
> (p. 38)

Levinson was a pioneer and trailblazer in the practice of CAC.

Over the past 50 years, the practice of CAC has continued to grow, with authors and researchers providing additional clarity and depth to the field of CAI. Like Levinson, there have been several pioneers in the practice of animal-assisted interactions (AAIs) in mental health. In his book *Handbook of Animal-Assisted Therapy*, Fine (2015) addressed important topics including the conceptualization of the human-animal bond, models and guidelines for quality assurance, best practices with special populations, and special topics and concerns in AAI. Contributing chapters in the special topics section include information on ensuring animal welfare, strategies for establishing an evidence base, and loss of a therapy animal.

In *Animal-Assisted Therapy in Counseling*, Chandler (2017) covered a wealth of topics including integrating AAI and counseling theories, crisis and disaster response, and international considerations for animal-assisted therapy (AAT). Chandler emphasized that to promote safety and reduce liability in the practice of animal-assisted counseling (AAC), practitioners should receive training with their animal partner, screen clients as a fit for AAC, review AAC-specific informed consent topics, understand how to prevent zoonoses, assess and respond to animal stress and welfare during sessions, establish clinical goals that incorporate AAC interventions, and assess client progress.

In her book on *Animal-Assisted Psychotherapy* (AAP), Parish-Plass (2013) presents AAP as a theory-based approach to working with clients. The book covers guiding principles, mechanisms, techniques, and dilemmas in the practice of AAP. There is a particular emphasis in this book on the triadic nature of AAP—the interaction and interplay between the therapist, client, and animal. All of these comprehensive contributions to the practice of AAC have deepened our knowledge and understanding of integrating animals into clinical practice. Together this work helps establish CAC as a distinct field requiring advanced training.

Several researchers have reported positive effects for CAC. In a study on including a dog in group counseling with teens, participants reported that the dog had a calming effect on group members, increased feelings of safety, and increased motivation to attend group sessions (Lange, Cox, Bernert, & Jenkins, 2006/2007). As mentioned in Chapter 2, Hartwig (2017) conducted a randomized comparison study that employed the Human-Animal Resilience Therapy (HART) intervention in individual counseling sessions with youths ages 10 to 18. The outcomes from this study revealed statistically significant decreases in anxiety, depression, and disruptive behavior scores for youths working with a therapy dog and youths working without a therapy dog in individual counseling. In a study involving youths in residential care who participated in counseling, Muela, Balluerka, Amiano, Caldentey, and Aliri (2017) indicated that participants in the animal-assisted group reported significant improvement in depression and sense of inadequacy when compared to control group participants. In a study on group counseling with children who had been sexually abused, Dietz, Davis, and Pennings (2012) found that children in the animal-assisted groups showed significant decreases in trauma symptoms, including anxiety, depression, anger, and dissociation.

Despite this evidence attesting to the benefits of CAC, there have been calls for more rigorous research. Hoagwood, Acri, Morrissey, and Peth-Pierce (2017) asserted that although there is some evidence of the positive effects of animal-assisted mental health services with youths, there needs to be more rigorous research to establish this modality as an evidence-based practice. In an effort to move the practice of animal-assisted mental health forward, Jones, Rice, and Cotton (2018) provided a series of recommendations for professionalizing the practice: use of consistent terms and definitions, development of manualized and theoretically grounded interventions, creation of clinical governance bodies and accreditation standards, and support for more clinical research. These recommendations provide helpful guidance for the next steps in CAC program and research development.

Practitioners Perspectives of AAC

An often-overlooked dimension of HAI research is investigating the views of the individuals at the heart of AAC: the practitioners. Hartwig and Smelser (2018) administered surveys to explore perspectives of mental health practitioners ($N = 343$) regarding the practice of AAC and the experience and training that is needed to effectively facilitate AAC with clients. The majority of practitioners who responded to the study (91.7%) indicated that they viewed AAC as a legitimate counseling modality. For clinical issues best addressed in AAC, respondents identified anxiety, depression, trauma, grief

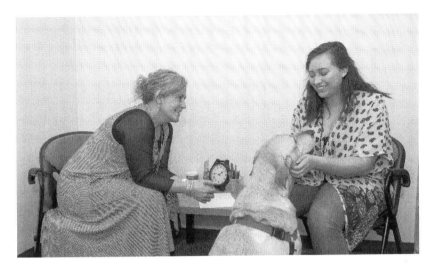

Figure 6.4 Professional counselor Mary Stone and therapy dog Wilson provide canine-assisted counseling to a teen client.

and loss, and abuse. Practitioners reported a wide client age range from 4 to 66 years and older as benefitting from AAC, with adolescents receiving the highest rate of responses (94.9%). An interesting finding in the study is that only one third of respondents reported being somewhat or very knowledgeable about AAC. Thus, the majority of participants did not have a working knowledge of the process, training, and standards for AAC. The findings from this study demonstrate the need to clarify and promote the training and standards required to optimally practice CAC.

Why Teams Need to Develop Competence in CAC

In our research on published criteria for therapy dog teams (Hartwig & Binfet, 2019), we identified that the training provided to CAI teams doing volunteer work is often absent or lacking. In turn, most volunteer CAI organizations do not provide sufficient or adequate training for teams working in clinical settings where nuanced and specialized interactions occur between practitioners, therapy dogs, and clients. In this section we'll present ethical codes and principles that inform and guide CAC training, describe the training required of mental health practitioners, and review AAC competencies.

Ethical Codes

In order to promote the integrity of the profession and ensure the well-being of clients, mental health practitioners are called to follow ethical codes. Because

Table 6.1 Ethical Codes Related to Competence in Mental Health Specialization Areas

Source	Code
American Association for Marriage and Family Therapy (AAMFT)	**3.6. Development of New Skills** "While developing new skills in specialty areas, marriage and family therapists take steps to ensure the competence of their work and to protect clients from possible harm. Marriage and family therapists practice in specialty areas new to them only after appropriate education, training, and/or supervised experience" (AAMFT, 2015, p. 5).
American Counseling Association (ACA)	**C.2.b. New Specialty Areas of Practice** "Counselors practice in specialty areas new to them only after appropriate education, training, and supervised experience. While developing skills in new specialty areas, counselors take steps to ensure the competence of their work and protect others from possible harm" (ACA, 2014, p. 8).
American Psychological Association (APA)	**2.01.c. Boundaries of Competence** "Psychologists planning to provide services, teach, or conduct research involving populations, areas, techniques, or technologies new to them undertake relevant education, training, supervised experience, consultation, or study" (APA, 2017, p. 5).
National Association of Social Workers (NASW)	**1.04.b. Competence** "Social workers should provide services in substantive areas or use intervention techniques or approaches that are new to them only after engaging in appropriate study, training, consultation, and supervision from people who are competent in those interventions or techniques" (NASW, 2017).

CAC is considered a specialization, we look to ethical codes to inform competence in specialization areas. Several ethical codes affirm the importance of developing competence in specialty areas of practice, such as CAC (see Table 6.1).

All of these ethical codes assert that mental health practitioners need *education, training, and supervised experience* in specialization areas. This means that practitioners interested in CAC need training and supervision in how to work with their dog in a clinical setting, not just training to work with their dog in a volunteer setting. We'll address these three processes of developing competence later in the chapter, but let's explore the ethical principles that govern mental health professionals next.

Ethical Principles

In addition to ethical codes, there are fundamental principles of professional ethical behavior. These ethical principles were established and are in place to guide practitioners' behavior and decision-making. The American Counseling Association (2014, p. 3) defines these principles as (a) autonomy, or "fostering the right to control the direction of one's life"; (b) nonmaleficence, or "avoiding actions that cause harm"; (c) beneficence, or "working for the good of the individual and society by promoting mental health and wellbeing"; (d) justice, or "treating individuals equitably and fostering fairness and equality"; (e) fidelity, or "honoring commitments and keeping promises, including fulfilling one's responsibilities of trust in professional relationships"; and (f) veracity, or "dealing truthfully with individuals with whom counselors come into professional contact." These ethical principles may have originally been designed uniquely for clinical work, yet these principles inform our understanding of how HAI is situated within the professional context of CAC. Table 6.2 presents an application of each ethical principle to CAC.

These principles provide a valuable foundation for working with dogs in counseling.

One of the principles, nonmaleficence, is addressed in both the AAMFT and ACA ethical codes related to competence in specialization areas. These two professional codes stress that practitioners must take steps to ensure competence so that clients are protected from possible harm. What kind of harm could occur in CAC? Examples of potential harm to clients in CAC include:

- client injury through a dog scratch, mouthing, or bite;
- discomfort with a dog due to cultural values;
- fear of the dog based on previous negative experiences with animals;
- anxiety related to unpredictability of dogs;
- medical concerns associated with allergies and animal-transmitted diseases; and
- feeling devalued based on disinterest in dog involvement in counseling.

Table 6.2 Ethical Principles Applied to Canine-Assisted Counseling

Ethical Principles	CAC Applications
Autonomy	Allowing the client to choose if he or she wants to work with a therapy dog
Nonmaleficence	Receiving training in CAC so the practitioners know how to avoid harm or injury to a client
Beneficence	Developing a client treatment plan that involves the dog, so that the dog is a part of promoting client progress in counseling
Justice	Allowing the dog to have a choice in how he or she wants to participate in the session
Fidelity	Bringing the dog to counseling when the practitioner says she or he will and explaining why the dog is not able to come on days when the dog cannot participate
Veracity	Reviewing and discussing an animal-assisted informed consent form to ensure that clients are fully informed prior to working with a dog in counseling

In addition to conceivable harm to clients, dogs can also be harmed in CAC. Examples of potential harm to dogs in CAC include:

- dog injury due to a client stepping, tripping, or pressing on parts of the dog's body;
- dog discomfort with client proximity, actions, or interventions that cause observable canine stress signals;
- medical concerns due to allergies or zoonoses; and
- dog demonstrating disinterest in engaging with clients or interventions as evidenced by turning, walking, sitting, or sleeping away from the client and session-related activities.

When practitioners want to involve a dog in counseling, it's important the practitioner learn how to protect the client *and* dog from harm. If the fundamental ethical values and principles assert that practitioners should receive education, training, and supervision in specialization areas and "do no harm" to clients, then it's not only important to follow these guidelines but also *unethical* if practitioners don't receive education, training, and supervision in CAC.

Mental Health Practitioner Training

There are several credentialing entities for mental health practitioner graduate programs. For the purpose of this chapter, we will use the Council for Accreditation of Counseling and Related Educational Programs (CACREP, 2018) as a framework for how mental health practitioners ought to be trained. CACREP provides national standards for counselor education programs through their accreditation process. CACREP currently accredits more than 870 graduate programs at 393 institutions across the United States (CACREP, 2018). CACREP's mission is to promote professional competence of counselors. CACREP standards offer a framework for the proficient training of mental health practitioners and serve as an example of how AAC training programs can model curricula. The 2016 CACREP standards required that counseling training programs integrate the following criteria:

- Students must receive education in eight core content areas and have a minimum of 60 semester credit hours of graduate-level education.
- Students must complete a 100-hour practicum, with 40 hours of direct client service (i.e., session with clients) and weekly supervision; students must also complete a 600-hour internship with a minimum of 240 hours of direct client service and weekly supervision.
- Faculty must systematically assess students' knowledge and skills throughout the program (CACREP, 2016).

The primary components of the CACREP standards include knowledge, practice, and assessment. As mental health practitioners and educators, we value the process used to train people to become effective counselors. This structure provides a helpful framework for CAC programs to use for the proficient and comprehensive training of practitioners and therapy dogs. This training structure also adheres to the ethical codes that indicate that practitioners interested in specialization areas must develop competence through education, training, and supervision.

AAT in Counseling Competencies

The CACREP standards lay the foundation for more specialized training in CAC. In order to develop training protocols in CAC, an understanding of competencies for working with animals in clinical contexts was needed. In 2016 the ACA endorsed animal-assisted therapy in counseling (AATC) competencies developed by Stewart, Chang, Parker, and Grubbs (2016). The AATC competencies are separated into three domains: knowledge, skills, and attitudes. The *knowledge* domain upholds that practitioners develop a comprehensive knowledge base of AAC history and evidence-based literature, foundations of HAI, animal physiology and care, noncoercive training techniques, canine stress signals, ethical requirements related to AAC, strategies for preventing harm, and infection prevention. The *skills* domain emphasizes that practitioners should have a strong foundation in basic counseling skills, consider AAC as a clinically intentional approach to helping clients, be able to incorporate theory-based AAC interventions, attend to both the client and animal concurrently, respond to animal stress and interactions with clients, and address animal care during sessions. The *attitudes* domain highlights that practitioners should promote animal welfare and advocacy, engage in professional development, and demonstrate the professional values of the AAC field. The competencies provide specific indicators for *knowledge*, *skills*, and *attitudes* and serve as published guidelines for practitioners interested in AAC.

CAC Training

As the interest in therapy dogs in clinical contexts increased and the AATC competencies emerged, the need for the development of training in CAC became essential. For many years, the only training offered for any form of CAI was provided by CAI organizations whose primary mission was to train volunteer CAI teams. As discussed in Chapter 5, CAI organizations that train volunteer teams provide no training or brief training, such as an online or 1-day training. This training may be a fit for teams who are providing short-term canine-assisted activities but does not meet competencies needed for longer term clinical services provided in mental health settings. The volunteer CAI organizations do not provide specialized training in the three AATC competency domains and in specific clinical skills, such as professional practice with clients, treatment planning, and CAC-focused supervision. Some AAI training programs offer online training that meets some of these competencies, such as knowledge about animal welfare, CAC interventions, and literature. However, these programs still do not offer live training and supervision of professional CAC practice with clients. In order for CAC programs to endorse practitioners to work in mental health settings with their dogs, and for practitioners to meet ethical standards, it's essential for practitioners to receive training and supervision in CAC prior to working with clients.

To respond to the need for specialized training in CAC, Dr. Hartwig developed the Texas State University Animal-Assisted Counseling Academy. The AAC Academy is one illustration of a training program that meets ethical standards for competency by teaching knowledge, clinical skills, professional practice, and supervision. The aim in presenting information about this training program is for potential CAC teams to evaluate and consider training programs that best meet ethical standards for competency in AAC. Next, we provide a history of the AAC Academy and an overview of the training protocol used to prepare teams for work as mental health practitioners.

In 2013 Dr. Hartwig developed curriculum for an animal-assisted training program at Texas State University for mental health practitioners and their dogs to participate in a study on CAC with youths ages 10 to 18. All of her study practitioners were required to become registered therapy dog teams through a CAI organization. They also participated in intensive AAC training that included AAC training for practitioners, preassessment for potential therapy dogs, preparation and practice for team evaluations, and then clinical practice with volunteer clients in the counseling clinic. Dr. Hartwig also developed a 10-week intervention curriculum, called the Human-Animal Resilience Therapy (HART) curriculum, for the study that provided guidelines and resources for 10 consecutive CAC interventions to utilize with clients in the study. After completing the study (see Hartwig, 2017, for more information on study outcomes), she expanded the training program, which then became the Texas State University Animal-Assisted Counseling (AAC) Academy. The AAC Academy began in 2016 and has graduated several cohorts of AAC teams since then. What follows are the steps to becoming credentialed through the AAC Academy.

Step 1: CAC Prerequisites

A prerequisite for the AAC Academy is that practitioners and their dogs must have a Canine Good Citizen (CGC) certificate prior to applying to the program. This is to ensure that both the practitioners and their dogs have mastered basic skills as a team and are ready for more advanced training in the CAC. This fits with our recommendation to utilize the CGC as a prerequisite for any CAI team training outlined in Chapter 5. Practitioners are required to upload their CGC certificate when they apply to the AAC Academy.

Step 2: Introduction to CAC

This is the first of three intensive trainings offered by the AAC Academy. Each training is composed of 4 days of training with prerequisite reading (e.g., typically books and articles) that must be completed prior to the beginning of the 4-day intensive. This first training only involves the practitioner (i.e., no dogs). This training provides an introduction to AAC and play therapy, history and theory of CAC, the practitioner-animal bond, evidence-based research in CAC, various therapeutic settings, canine communication, and positive training approaches for CAC. During this training, AAC Academy graduates come to the university with their therapy dogs to share with participants information and insights about their work in private practice, school, and clinical settings. After this training, practitioners schedule time with Dr. Hartwig for a preassessment with their dog. All dogs are pre-assessed prior to being allowed on campus, even if they have already passed the CGC test. This is an additional layer of screening for the CAC team evaluation to ensure that the therapy dogs will be a good fit for being on campus and around other dogs during the next two AAC Academy trainings.

Step 3: Intermediate Methods in CAC

This is the second of three intensive trainings offered by the AAC Academy. This training provides intermediate training in AAC and play therapy skills and techniques in the context of a practitioner-animal team. Practitioners bring their dogs to this training, along with a crate, toys, treats, and water bowls. Dogs are spaced out in the classroom, are not allowed to interact with other dogs, and must remain leashed and with their practitioner partner at all times. In this training, Dr. Hartwig teaches practitioners various CAC interventions that they can employ with clients with different clinical goals and developmental needs. Because the AAC Academy provides continuing education credits for play therapy, practitioners also learn about play therapy and working with children and canines together. Another key component of this training is skill learning and practice for the AAC team evaluation. Just as we encouraged CAI teams to practice evaluation skills in Chapter 5, we believe that CAC teams should practice skills for the AAC team evaluation prior to being evaluated. At the end of this training, we schedule teams for the AAC team evaluation.

Step 4: CAC Team Evaluation

The CAC team evaluation is an in-person assessment of how the practitioner works with their canine partner in a counseling setting. Practitioners and the canine partners must pass the CAC team evaluation prior to moving on to the Practicum in CAC training and working with clients. The CAC team evaluation is similar to the CAI team assessment that we'll cover next in Chapter 7, with several additional skills that focus on clinical work with clients and dogs. As the CAC team evaluation is being prepared for publication, readers are encouraged to look for its published version soon.

Step 5: Practicum in CAC

This is the third of three trainings offered by the AAC Academy and is the culmination of all the learning that teams have gained throughout the AAC Academy. This training for teams is composed of a practicum that provides advanced training in CAC and play therapy facilitative skills and techniques through supervision that sees CAC teams working with clients. Practitioners also bring their dogs to this training. The primary aim of the practicum training is to provide live professional practice with volunteer clients in a clinical setting. Each CAC team facilitates four sessions with clients during the practicum. Teams are supervised by Dr. Hartwig, peers, and other clinical supervisors. While CAC teams are in sessions, observers complete the CAC Skills Checklist, which is covered in the next section. This checklist lists skills that CAC teams should demonstrate during the session. After CAC teams complete their counseling sessions, the teams participate in both group and individual supervision. CAC teams share their perspectives about the sessions and discuss case conceptualizations. Observers share strengths and areas of

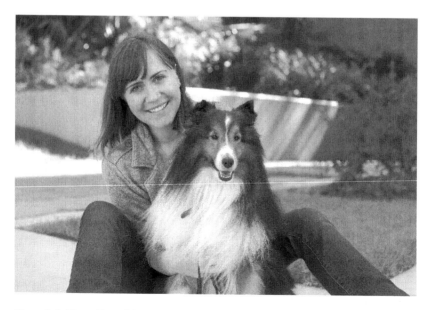

Figure 6.5 Texas State University Animal-Assisted Counseling Academy graduates Allison Desjardins and Cooper.

growth for each session, based on their notes from the CAC Skills Checklist. This live professional practice and supervision process is integral to how CAC teams learn and develop clinical skills in partnership with their therapy dog.

Step 6: Supervision in CAC

After the Practicum in CAC training, practitioners must facilitate 100 hours of CAC with their therapy dog while receiving supervision. CAC supervision provides practitioners with posttraining support and guidance. This allows practitioners the opportunity to enhance and hone their CAC skills in their own clinical settings. CAC supervision is provided by Dr. Hartwig in an encrypted online format that is compliant with the Health Insurance Portability and Accountability Act of 1996 (HIPAA). The 10 supervision sessions include case consultation, CAC skills assessment, ethical decision-making discussions, CAC technique sharing, and treatment planning. Practitioners track CAC hours and supervision on a spreadsheet provided by the AAC Academy.

Step 7: Certification and Recertification

Once practitioners have met all program requirements, they submit their CAC hours and supervision spreadsheet. They then receive a certificate for professional credentialing in CAC. This certificate is endorsed by Texas State University.

CAC Skills Checklist

In order for participants to develop effective skills, it's important for them to know the specific skills they need to develop. Dr. Hartwig developed the CAC Skills Checklist as a tool for CAC supervisors, practitioners, and peers to use in order to ensure that practitioners are clear on their strengths and areas of growth in developing each skill. This checklist is used in the AAC Academy for each live counseling session that a practitioner facilitates during CAC practicum with a client. CAC supervisors and peers observe sessions live and complete the checklist while they are watching the session. It's important to acknowledge that many of the skills on this checklist are not taught as part of the training provided by volunteer CAI organizations. These are skills that CAC practitioners should be able to demonstrate for the well-being of clients and canine partners, but practitioners often don't receive training, practice, or supervision on these skills unless they participate in an AAI mental health training program that incorporates a practicum component into their training.

For this section we will provide the name of each skill, a description of the skill, and an explanation for why this skill is important for clinical work with dogs. This form is available in **Appendix C.**

Preliminary Skills

Preliminary skills are skills that the practitioner demonstrates at the beginning of the session. These skills are important because they establish that the practitioner is prepared, is ensuring and safeguarding the client's and dog's welfare, and supports a positive transition from presession to the working part of the session.

1. Skill name: **Appearance and grooming**

   Skill description: The practitioner is dressed appropriately for CAC sessions. The dog was bathed and groomed prior to session.

   Why it's important in CAC: Practitioners and dogs should be well groomed and have a professional appearance for clinical work with a client. Dogs need to be bathed in order to avoid activating allergies in clients.

2. Skill name: **Hygiene**

   Skill description: The practitioner asks the client to wash hands or use hand sanitizer prior to touching the dog.

   Why it's important in CAC: Handwashing can help reduce human- and canine-transmitted diseases.

3. Skill name: **Greeting the dog**

   Skill description: The practitioner shows the client how to greet the dog prior to the client meeting the dog. The practitioner guides the greeting interaction between the client and dog.

   Why it's important in CAC: Many people don't know how to greet a dog in the way that a dog likes to be greeted. Teaching clients and family members how to greet a dog in counseling should be a consistent practice for first sessions.

4. Skill name: **Dog bonding time**

   Skill description: The practitioner begins the session with at least 5 minutes of client and dog bonding time.

   Why it's important in CAC: Dog bonding time allows for relationship building between the client, dog, and counselor at the beginning of the session. It also provides the client and dog with time to transition from presession activities (e.g., running to make the appointment on time) to session interventions.

5. Skill name: **Teaching canine communication**

   Skill description: The practitioner teaches the client about species-specific canine communication skills during the session.

   Why it's important in CAC: As clients and dog are together for a longer time frame than typical CAIs, teaching the client how to identify and recognize behavioral indicators that show canine stress or contentment is crucial in counseling. This allows the client to have an understanding of what the dog is communicating (e.g., if the dog enjoys or is tolerating a certain interaction).

6. Skill name: **Canine welfare**

   Skill description: The practitioner ensures that the dog is healthy and well rested, has access to fresh water, and receives a break each hour.

   Why it's important in CAC: Chapter 4 addressed components of ensuring canine welfare. In CAC, practitioners are responsible for ensuring that dogs have gone to the bathroom before sessions, have access to fresh water, receive breaks after each session, and are not being asked to do more they can do within a particular session and over the course of a working day or week. As there is currently no limit to the number of hours a dog can participate in CAC sessions, practitioners should pay attention to the energy level of their dog and limit sessions based on canine behavior and communication.

Facilitative and Advanced Skills

Facilitative skills are also referred to as basic counseling skills in mental health fields. These skills are the foundation for all counseling skills, even prior to integrating a theoretical approach. Facilitative skills show the client that the

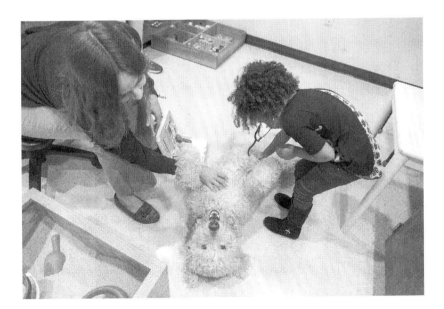

Figure 6.6 A child client checks therapy dog Cash as part of a canine-assisted play therapy session with practitioner Jillian Zuboy.

practitioner is listening, acknowledging feelings, and grasping the meaning of the client's words and the dog's behavior. In addition to these basic skills, there are other skills in this section that are more advanced, such as limit setting and facilitating the client-dog relationship. These advanced skills promote the human-canine bond and client and dog safety.

1. Skill name: **Reflection of nonverbal behavior (i.e., tracking)**

   Skill description: The practitioner demonstrates reflection of nonverbal behavior in relation to CAC interactions.

   Why it's important in CAC: This skill allows the practitioner to acknowledge what the client or dog is doing in the session. If the dog is offering a behavior, such as wanting to sit by the client, and the client doesn't respond, this is an example of how reflecting what the dog is doing could be helpful.

2. Skill name: **Reflection of content**

   Skill description: The practitioner demonstrates reflection of verbal content in relation to CAC interactions.

   Why it's important in CAC: Reflecting content allows the practitioner to acknowledge what the client or dog is saying or potentially communicating in the session. Sometimes counselors use the phrase, "So what I hear you saying . . ." as a way to reflect content. For reflecting dog content, some CAC practitioners choose to reflect what they think a dog is saying or thinking and others don't (e.g., "Chango's not sure what he thinks about that toy.").

3. Skill name: **Reflection of feeling**

   Skill description: The practitioner demonstrates reflection of feeling in relation to CAC interactions.

   Why it's important in CAC: Reflecting feeling allows the practitioner to acknowledge what the client or dog is feeling in the session. This is an important skill because it can help clients make connections between their feelings and thoughts or behaviors. CAC practitioners should also use this skill to facilitate how the client feels about client-dog interactions.

4. Skill name: **Nonverbal skills**

   Skill description: The practitioner demonstrates effective use of head, eyes, hands, feet, posture, and voice with client and dog.

   Why it's important in CAC: Nonverbal skills show that the practitioner is positioned, moves, and speaks in a way that promotes the therapeutic alliance. These skills are helpful for practitioner interactions with the client (e.g., appearing open by not crossing arms and legs) and the dog (e.g., not holding the dog tightly or scolding the dog).

5.   Skill name: **Empathy**

Skill description: The practitioner communicates empathy, respect, and unconditional positive regard to client and dog.

Why it's important in CAC: Empathy, respect, and unconditional positive regard compose Rogers's (1980) core components in counseling. CAC practitioners should be able to demonstrate these core components to both the client and the dog.

6.   Skill name: **Client-canine relationship**

Skill description: The practitioner demonstrates facilitation of the client-canine relationship so that a working alliance is developed.

Why it's important in CAC: An important element of CAC sessions is the development of the client-dog relationship. The practitioner must be able to demonstrate the facilitation of the relationship from the beginning of the session to the end. The practitioner can do this by acknowledging "relational moments" (Chandler, 2017) between the client and dog, or by using facilitation skills ("Riley really wants you to throw the ball to him.").

7.   Skill name: **Questions**

Skill description: The practitioner demonstrates appropriate use of open-ended and close-ended questions, with an emphasis on open-ended questions.

Why it's important in CAC: Practitioners should be able to demonstrate a balance between purposeful questions and facilitative skills. The overuse of questions can be overwhelming for clients. The use of open-ended questions (i.e., questions that start with "what" or "how") allows clients to answer in a variety of ways as compared to close-ended questions, in which the client is able to answer with a yes or no. Questions used in CAC should also involve questions about the client-dog relationship and interactions.

8.   Skill name: **Limit setting**

Skill description: The practitioner sets limits with the client or dog as needed to promote positive practitioner-canine interaction. The practitioner redirects the client or dog immediately when the dog shows stress signals. The practitioner discusses reasons for limit setting or redirection in relation to the human-canine bond.

Why it's important in CAC: Chapter 5 presented the concept of limit setting through Landreth's (2012) ACT model. Setting boundaries and limits is an important skill for practitioners in CAC because sometimes clients or dogs may need redirecting. Setting limits has the potential to prevent or alleviate negative interactions, canine stress, or injury.

9. Skill name: **Client-canine communication and response**

   Skill description: The practitioner observes the client and dog through-out session for stress signals and responds immediately to reduce client or canine stress and promote safety.

   Why it's important in CAC: Practitioners should be fluent in interpreting canine communication and behavior. In sessions, practitioners should recognize stress in the client or their dog and respond immediately. For example, "Grace, I notice you're uncomfortable with Holly sitting next to you right now. Holly, come sit over here. Good girl!" For another example, "Thomas, I can see that you enjoy patting Wilson on the head, but I notice Wilson puts his head down and closes his mouth each time you do that. He's communicating that he doesn't like that. Let's try stroking his back and see if he likes that."

10. Skill name: **Canine-specific boundaries**

    Skill description: The practitioner ensures that the dog participates in ways that are safe and comfortable for the dog. The dog is allowed to choose to participate or not during the session.

    Why it's important in CAC: One of the most important values in a CAC session is that the dog is permitted to participate in the ways that she or he likes. This means that if a dog doesn't want to sit by a client, receive petting, or be involved in an intervention, that's fine and is allowed. The dog can choose to be involved or not. Dogs should always have a place where they can go if they choose to not be involved in the session.

11. Skill name: **Confidence**

    Skill description: The practitioner demonstrates appropriate levels of self-assurance and trust in own ability and dog's ability.

    Why it's important in CAC: CAC practitioners need to have confidence in their clinical abilities and in their ability to work with both a client (or clients) and a dog at the same time. If a practitioner feels uncertain about their CAC skills, they should seek out additional supervision and practice opportunities.

Next, we'll examine the more focused skills of therapeutic intentionality. In CAC, these clinical skills must also integrate the dog into the practitioner's work with the client.

Therapeutic Intentionality Skills

This section is composed of skills that demonstrate a practitioner's ability to integrate CAC into other elements of clinical work, such as goal setting, the use of clinical theory, the employment of CAC interventions, and intentionality.

1. Skill name: **Goal setting**

   Skill description: The practitioner collaborates with the client to establish realistic and measurable goals that address the presenting problem and integrate the dog and CAC techniques.

   Why it's important in CAC: Involving a dog in a session should be purposeful. In counseling, clients should set measurable goals that are then added to a treatment plan. The integration of a dog should be a part of the treatment plan that helps the client work toward the goal they set for counseling. If a dog would not support a client in working toward their goal (e.g., the client has a fear of dogs and does not want to work on that in counseling), then the dog should not be involved in sessions with the client.

2. Skill name: **Theory**

   Skill description: The practitioner demonstrates understanding and appropriate application of a counseling theory as part of CAC.

   Why it's important in CAC: Practitioners should use a theoretical framework to guide their work with clients.

3. Skill name: **Interventions**

   Skill description: The practitioner utilizes and develops CAC interventions that integrate the dog into the therapeutic process.

   Why it's important in CAC: One of the main reasons for incorporating a dog into counseling is for the dog to be a part of the client's progress toward clinical goals. The dog can be involved in interactive interventions, such as the Thumball™ intervention in the opening scenario, or passive interventions, such as sitting next to a client and providing comfort. When developing a client's treatment plan, the practitioner should plan interventions that involve the dog in supporting client goals.

4. Skill name: **Intentionality**

   Skill description: The practitioner demonstrates a clear understanding of therapeutic intention using theory and CAC interventions to work toward clinical goals.

   Why it's important in CAC: Intentionality can be observed through the integration of how the practitioners connects the involvement of the dog with clinical theory and CAC interventions that support client goals. This skill is more of an overall impression of bringing several skills together. This skill can also be observed in case consultation and supervision after the session.

CAC Skills Checklist Rating

The checklist includes a column for rating each of these skills. The purpose of the ratings is not to have an overall score, but rather to assess each skill and identify skills that are strengths for the practitioner and areas for growth. The ratings for each skill are:

- N: Not applicable/no opportunity to observe;
- O: Does not demonstrate this skill;
- 1: Demonstrates this skill minimally;
- 2: Demonstrates this skill variably; and
- 3: Demonstrates this skill consistently.

There is also a column for comments. In this column, observers can write examples of how the skills were demonstrated (e.g., client-canine relationship: "You acknowledged that Korra sat close to the client and processed how the client felt about that."), positive feedback (e.g., dog bonding time: "Great bonding activity! Both the client and Manny enjoyed finding and answering the questions on the tennis balls."), or constructive comments (e.g., limit setting: "The client got too close to Coco's face during the mindfulness intervention. In the future, you need to intervene faster and set a limit."). In addition to the rating and comments columns, the checklist has an additional page to write overall strengths and areas for growth. This provides space to provide overall feedback, such as how the practitioner handled an ethical dilemma, suggestions for applying theoretical techniques that involve the dog, and recommendations for future interventions with the client.

Conclusion

This chapter explored the practice and training required for CAC. In the beginning of the chapter, we provided an overview of CAC literature and a discussion of why CAC teams need to develop competence. We then presented a training framework for CAC that meets ethical standards for developing competence in a specialized field. Last, we provided a description of the CAC Skills Checklist that can be used to assess practitioner skills for CAC sessions. In the next chapter we'll delve into CAI team assessment.

References

American Association for Marriage and Family Therapy (AAMFT). (2015). *Code of ethics.* Retrieved from www.aamft.org/Legal_Ethics/Code_of_Ethics.aspx

American Counseling Association (ACA). (2014). *ACA code of ethics.* Retrieved from www.counseling.org/resources/aca-code-of-ethics.pdf

American Psychological Association (APA). (2017). *Ethical principles of psychologists and code of conduct.* Retrieved from www.apa.org/ethics/code/ethics-code-2017.pdf

Chandler, C. K. (2017). *Animal assisted therapy in counseling* (3rd ed.). New York: Routledge.

Council for Accreditation of Counseling and Related Educational Programs (CACREP). (2016). *2016 CACREP standards.* Retrieved from www.cacrep.org/wp-content/uploads/2018/05/2016-Standards-with-Glossary-5.3.2018.pdf

Council for Accreditation of Counseling and Related Educational Programs (CACREP). (2018). *Annual report 2017*. Alexandria, VA: CACREP.

Dietz, T. J., Davis, D., & Pennings, J. (2012). Evaluating animal-assisted therapy in group treatment for child sexual abuse. *Journal of Child Sexual Abuse*, 21(6), 665–683. doi: 10.1080/10538712.2012.726700.

Fine, A. H. (Ed.) (2015). *Handbook of animal-assisted therapy: Foundations and guidelines for animal-assisted interventions* (4th ed.). San Diego, CA: Academic Press.

Hartwig, E. K. (2017). Building solutions in youth: Evaluation of the Human-Animal Resilience Therapy intervention. *Journal of Creativity in Mental Health*, 12(4), 468–481. doi: 10.1080/15401383.2017.1283281.

Hartwig, E. K., & Binfet, J. T. (2019). What's important in canine-assisted intervention teams? An investigation of canine-assisted intervention program online screening tools. *Journal of Veterinary Behavior: Clinical Applications and Research*, 29, 53–60.

Hartwig, E. K., & Smelser, Q. K. (2018). Practitioner perspectives on animal-assisted counseling. *Journal of Mental Health Counseling*, 40(1), 43–57. doi: 10.17744/mehc.40.1.04.

Hoagwood, K. E., Acri, M., Morrissey, M., & Peth-Pierce, R. (2017). Animal-assisted therapies for youth with or at risk for mental health problems: A systematic review. *Applied Developmental Science*, 21(1), 1–13. doi: 10.1080/10888691.2015.1134267.

Jones, M. G., Rice, S. M., & Cotton, S. M. (2018). Who let the dogs out? therapy dogs in clinical practice. *Australasian Psychiatry*, 26(2), 196–199. doi: 10.1177/10398562 17749056.

Lange, A., Cox, J., Bernert, D., & Jenkins, C. (2006/2007). Is counseling going to the dogs? An exploratory study related to the inclusion of an animal in group counseling with adolescents. *Journal of Creativity in Mental Health*, 2, 17–31. doi: 10.1300/J456v02n02_03.

Landreth, G. (2012). *Play therapy: The art of the relationship* (3rd ed.). New York: Brunner Routledge.

Levinson, B. (1969). *Pet-oriented child psychotherapy*. Springfield, IL: Charles C. Thomas, Bannerstone House.

National Association of Social Workers (NASW). (2017). *Code of ethics*. Retrieved from www.socialworkers.org/About/Ethics/Code-of-Ethics/Code-of-Ethics-English.

Muela, A., Balluerka, N., Amiano, N., Caldentey, M. A., & Aliri, J. (2017). Animal-assisted psychotherapy for young people with behavioural problems in residential care. *Clinical Psychology & Psychotherapy*, 24(6), 01484–01494. doi: 10.1002/cpp.2112.

Parish-Plass, N. (2013). *Animal-assisted psychotherapy: Theory, issues, and practice*. West Lafayette, IN: Purdue University Press.

Rogers, C. R. (1980). *A way of being*. Boston, MA: Houghton Mifflin.

Stewart, L. A., Chang, C. Y., Parker, L. K., & Grubbs, N. (2016). *Animal-assisted therapy in counseling competencies*. Alexandria, VA: American Counseling Association, Animal-Assisted Therapy in Mental Health Interest Network. Retrieved from www.counseling.org/docs/default-source/competencies/animal-assisted-therapy-competencies-june-2016.pdf?sfvrsn=14.

7 Canine-Assisted Intervention Team Assessment

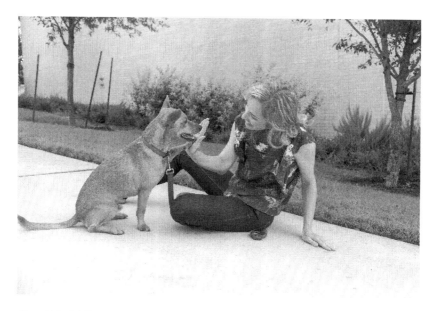

Figure 7.1 CAC practitioner Nicole Lozo and her therapy dog, Andy, make a great team.

In order to ensure that teams are well suited to and well prepared for CAI work and present no danger to the public, there is a need for prospective CAI teams to be comprehensively assessed. If our goal is to produce well-trained teams who can thrive in different settings, it's essential to determine the extent to which these teams are ready to work with clients. CAI assessments are complex because teams must work within varied settings with varied CAI clients and support their varied well-being goals. Together, these factors make developing a comprehensive CAI team assessment challenging. Butler (2013) asserts, "Human capacity to realistically assess the environments in which dogs are being required to work, and to respond ethically to what the dogs are communicating, must catch up with these new expectations being placed

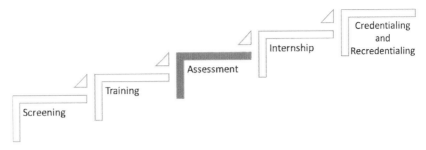

Figure 7.2 CAI team credentialing process.

upon the dogs" (Chapter 1, para. 14). As we begin this chapter, consider the following scenario.

Scenario

Jacob is excited to become credentialed as a CAI team with his dog, Lion, but is nervous about the assessment. The evaluator sent an e-mail a few days prior reminding him about the materials he'd need to bring, acceptable clothing and footwear, and approved collar and leash types. He hopes he has brought everything he needs for the assessment. When the evaluator greets him, Jacob shakes her hand and smiles. Lion is wagging his tail but does not approach or jump on the evaluator. Jacob enters the assessment room with Lion and they notice a few volunteers quietly talking, seated in chairs on one side of the room. The evaluator encourages Jacob to advocate for Lion throughout the assessment. The evaluator reminds Jacob that he and Lion have trained for this and practiced all of these skills several times over the past few months. Jacob bends down near Lion and tells him, "OK, Lion, let's do this!"

Questions for Reflection and Discussion

1. What can CAI organizations do to support teams like Jacob and Lion before, during, and after the CAI team assessment?
2. What skills do Jacob and Lion need to demonstrate for the assessment?
3. What behavioral indicators will the evaluator be looking for in order to score each team skill in the assessment?

In this chapter we'll delve into the complexities of CAI assessments with the goal of providing concrete recommendations for assessing both handlers and their dogs seeking to become credentialed CAI teams. We'll begin by exploring the challenges in assessing CAI teams, the current practices in CAI assessments, and how to prepare for a team assessment. Next, we'll provide a description of each assessment skill along with scoring guidelines and a provide a rationale illustrating why each skill is important. We'll end this chapter on assessing CAI teams with a review of assessment outcomes and a look beyond at what teams might expect once they're credentialed.

Why Assessment Is Important

As Figure 7.2 illustrated, there is a progression that prospective teams follow that begins with CAI organizations screening potential teams (recall our Screening Intake Form discussed in Chapter 1) and then offering training to teams so they are the prepared for the CAI team assessment that follows. The comprehensive assessment of CAI teams is important for three reasons. First, assessing prospective teams helps to ensure public safety. We have all heard stories of poorly trained or managed dogs misbehaving or even being aggressive when out in public. The work asked of a credentialed CAI team is very public in nature, and if our primary goal in providing CAI to clients is to promote their well-being, then we have to ensure that CAI teams do not cause harm. Second, assessing teams is important as it ensures that teams are qualified and capable and have the skills needed to promote client well-being for the client population they support and for the context in which they work. The assessment of teams helps ensure that the team is prepared to work in the context for which they have been trained. If a CAI team plans to work with children, then that team should be assessed around a child or children. And third, a comprehensive CAI team assessment ensures that HAIs are enjoyable for all stakeholders, that CAI organizations have strong teams volunteering or working on their behalf that allow them to fulfill their mission, and that the CAI teams themselves have a meaningful and enjoyable experience. All of these are important considerations in both the training and assessment of CAI teams.

Purpose and Challenges of the CAI Team Assessment

All CAI organizations should be committed to the comprehensive assessment of CAI team competence from the moment a prospective team completes a screening application to their being credentialed by an organization. CAI organizations have several responsibilities when conducting their team assessment.

Assess for Service Delivery

A key responsibility in the team assessment is the extent to which the assessment supports and reflects the skills that are needed for the facilities, clients, and degree of interaction. If teams will be required to be around medical equipment, then they should be assessed around medical equipment. If teams will be listening to a child reading, then the skills assessed in the assessment should match the complexities found within that interaction and that setting. Fredrickson-MacNamara and Butler (2010) note that few team assessments involve an assessment of skills with children, yet many teams are involved in programs with children. This is a dangerous practice, as children are still learning skills for impulse control and can be unpredictable around dogs. One of the best ways to develop assessments for service delivery is to ensure that handlers are prepared to support their canine partner in different contexts and especially when issues arise.

Assess for Diversity

Another key responsibility in the assessment of CAI teams is the extent to which the assessment takes into account aspects of diversity. As we discussed in Chapter 4, it's essential that CAI teams are prepared for working with diverse CAI clients in varied settings. This is especially important when teams are working public settings where the client is not predetermined (e.g., an airport or college campus). Such interactions require the handlers to recognize, assess, and respond to the cultural values of clients. Handler's must be aware that people differ in the value they accord animals (i.e., their beliefs around dogs in public venues) and that some people are fearful around dogs. Teaching handlers about the importance of asking clients if they would like to interact with a therapy dogs and asking handlers to be culturally sensitive helps ensure optimal canine-client interactions. The assessment of teams should incorporate gauging the dog's response to people of different ages, sex, sizes, skin colors, facial hair, and clothing (Binfet & Struik, 2018). If dogs are only assessed around people of a certain age, sex, or ethnicity, then organizations haven't fully guaranteed the dog will be safe when interacting with diverse clients. In Chapter 8 we explore nuanced assessment considerations

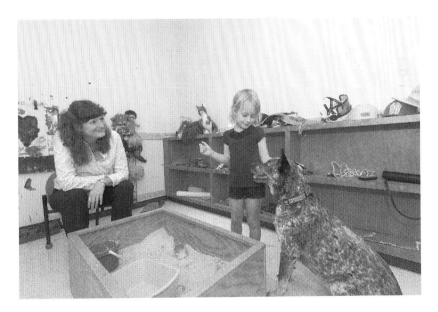

Figure 7.3 Canine-assisted play therapy with CAC practitioner Kim Sullivan and therapy dog Gordon.

for specialized contexts, such as medical or health care settings, airports, and college campuses.

The assessment of CAI team skills and dispositions is a challenging undertaking. Many published canine temperament and behavioral measures neglect to account for reliability, validity, and feasibility outcomes (Jones & Gosling, 2005; Taylor & Mills, 2006). That is, the psychometric properties (i.e., the extent to which the measures assess what they claim to assess and do so consistently across dogs and across varied contexts) can be problematic. Added to this, CAI organizations, many of whom are run by volunteers, can struggle with the capacity, funding, and resources required to conduct comprehensive assessments. Some of the capacity challenges organizations can face include training and maintaining trainers and evaluators, providing in-person training and support to teams throughout their geographic area, and procuring funding to support staff who coordinate these programs. As CAI organizations strive to develop screening, training, and assessment protocols to identify CAI teams to work on their behalf, consideration must be given to these capacity challenges.

An Overview of CAI Organization Assessments

A strategic way to understand CAI assessments is to explore the practices used throughout the broader CAI community around identifying CAI teams. The dynamic field of CAIs owes thanks to the pioneering work of several distinct movements or organizations who informed our thinking and initiated practices around how best to identify CAI teams. In Chapter 5 we presented the Canine Good Citizen (CGC) test developed by the American Kennel Club (AKC, 2018) as an example of a tool that CAI organizations can use as a prerequisite or screening device for CAI training. The CGC test was originally used as a behavioral indicator to support family dogs having good manners in the home and community and should continue to be used in the way that it was designed and intended. One key impact the CGC test had on the CAI field is in providing a foundational test from which other CAI team assessments were modeled or, at the very least, are similar. In the next section we present an overview of the assessment practices of three large CAI organizations.

First, Therapy Dogs International (TDI) was founded in 1976 by Elaine Smith, a registered nurse (TDI, 2019). TDI adapted the CGC test to include skills that more closely resembled a visit to a facility, such as including a skill for checking into the facility (Butler, 2013). Similar to CGC, there are no training requirements for handlers or dogs. TDI (2019) divides their assessment into two distinct phases: in Phase I, an evaluator assesses skills within a group context where multiple teams are present, and in Phase II, each individual team has their skills assessed. By requiring teams to be in the presence of other teams, TDI evaluators are able to determine how dogs respond when other dogs are nearby. The TDI assessment includes skills that are beneficial for volunteering in a facility, such as the skills required when visiting a patient, entering through a door at a facility, and the dog's reaction to children. TDI requires that teams be evaluated once.

Second, Pet Partners (2019) was originally founded in 1977 as the Delta Society®. Pet Partners developed their Therapy Animal Program in 1990. As can be seen on the Pet Partners website (2019), handlers interested in volunteering with Pet Partners must complete a 1-day or online handler training prior to being assessed as a team. According to Butler (2013), the Pet Partners assessment includes a skills test similar to the AKC's CGC test and also includes an aptitude test that is composed of skills to assess potential issues encountered on visits, such as clumsy petting, a restraining hug, and angry yelling. In addition to requiring handler training and an assessment that evaluates both skills and aptitude, Pet Partners requires teams to be reevaluated and to reregister every 2 years.

Third, Alliance of Therapy Dogs (ATD, 2019) was founded in 1990 and originally incorporated as Therapy Dogs Incorporated (TDInc.). In 2015 TDInc. changed their name to ATD. The requirements for ATD teams include one team assessment and three facility visits that are observed by a current ATD handler. Butler (2013) notes that observing teams is a beneficial step in assessing how teams may function in a facility. ATD requires a background check for volunteer CAI teams and an ATD rules review. The rules review asks for potential ATD handlers to discuss guidelines that are detailed in the ATD rules and regulations, such as "When does a visit begin and end?" (as soon as a team reaches the facility property and leaves the facility property; *ATD*, 2019). ATD does not have training requirements for handlers or dogs.

The assessment practices of these large therapy animal organizations contribute enormously to our understanding of just what is required to comprehensively evaluate prospective CAI teams. In addition to these large organizations, there are countless regional and community-based CAI organizations throughout the world. Some of these programs are affiliates of larger CAI organizations (e.g., Pet Partners of Central Texas), but many are established as their own, independent CAI organization complete with a specific mission, board of directors, and team credentialing requirements. The assessment practices and processes vary greatly among these organizations, from the basic requirement of merely having a friendly dog to organizations that evaluate 20 or more skills and require supervised visits.

Adding complexity and perhaps confusion to the assessment of CAI teams is the formation or training of the individuals at the helm of all of these varied organizations. Fredrickson-MacNamara and Butler (2010) argue that many CAI organizations were established in the 1990s by pet owners rather than professionals with formal training in HAI. Thus, lay people with wide-ranging training and experience, in turn, developed screening and assessment procedures to identify CAI teams. This resulted in ample variability within the field, and this inconsistency across organizations around the assessment of teams contributes to confusion among potential volunteers in knowing just what skills they need to become credentialed. Certainly, one of our aims in writing this book was to reduce some of this variability through our screening, training, and assessment model of credentialing CAI teams. Next, we identify and describe the conditions and skills contributing to the CAI team assessment.

Setting Up the Assessment Environment

Assuring that the assessment environment is organized, equipped, and safe helps create optimal conditions in which teams can showcase their skills and dispositions. Three environmental elements should be considered: (1) the room setup, (2) the volunteers, and (3) the stress level. The room should be reserved ahead of time and limited only to teams who are being assessed. As teams are evaluated individually, we recommend having both a waiting room and a room in which assessments are conducted. It's important that teams who have not yet been assessed do not interact with one another as a dog may react unpredictably or become stressed in the presence of other dogs.

Room Setup

In consideration of room size, rooms that are too large may intimidate teams, but rooms that are too small may not allow enough room for teams to demonstrate skills. Flooring may be a consideration in choosing a room for CAI team assessments. Some dogs are not used to walking on slippery surfaces, such as tile, linoleum, or laminate floors. Conducting assessments in a carpeted room is an option, but note that some dogs may be overly stressed during the assessment and eliminate on the floor. Another option is to provide a mat or allow teams to bring a mat or blanket from home.

Binfet and Struik (2018) recommend setting up stations for each skill with mats and resources prepared at each station. For example, a skill that requires a team to walk in an L-shape could use tape on the floor to mark the path to clarify expectations for teams. This prevents confusion and helps reduce stress in teams and supports them in the successful completion of each skill. Resources, such as long leashes, wheelchairs, walkers, robes, and hats, should be placed where they will be needed within the room to assist the evaluators and team is adjudicating and completing tasks. The room should be set up logically with skills sequenced so that safety is guaranteed.

Volunteers

Volunteers are vital to the success of the assessment, and CAI organizations would be wise to recruit volunteers from within their organization. This way, volunteers share the evaluator's mission and understanding of the process about to unfold. Prior to the assessment day, volunteers should be trained in the role they are serving and given an opportunity to practice skills as needed. What follows are the varied volunteer roles that contribute to a successful CAI team assessment:

- Check-in volunteer: This volunteer greets teams outside the assessment room, collects paperwork, ensures that teams wear nametags, and shows each team to the waiting room.
- Team evaluators: Evaluators facilitate the assessment and work collaboratively to review outcomes. It's helpful to have at least two evaluators to assess a potential CAI team.
- Assessment volunteers: These volunteers can play roles that help the evaluators assess the different skills required of the team. Several skills require at least three volunteers, so it's important to have enough volunteers to fulfill all of the specific roles required as part of the assessment. Ideally volunteers include people of different ages, genders, and skin tones, so that dogs can be assessed in their interactions with diverse clients. If teams will potentially be working with children, then there should be a child volunteer between the ages of 6 and 12 who can participate in some of the skills. All volunteers should practice their roles and script prior to the start of an assessment to reduce confusion.
- Neutral dog team: The neutral dog team is only present for the *reaction to a neutral dog* skill. The neutral dog team should be a credentialed team within the organization. Be mindful of how much is asked of neutral dog teams and where assessments are conducted over the course of a day, several teams should be booked to avoid overtaxing individual teams.

Reducing Stress Level

Handlers may be anxious about the assessment. This may be due to their passionate interest in passing the assessment, as this is the key to them serving as a CAI team. Handlers may be worried that their dog will not execute the skills correctly or after one cue or prompting. They may also be nervous at the idea of being watched by evaluators and volunteers. When handlers are stressed, this may potentially impact the stress level of their dog. There are several things that organizations and evaluators can do to reduce the stress level of handlers:

- Offer practice assessments: One of the best ways for people to learn skills is through practice. In many fields of study, students practice skills prior to ever working with clients, performing, or serving others (e.g., think about the benefits of dress rehearsals for theater performances). Similarly, giving teams the opportunity to practice running through the various assessment skills can be immensely encouraging. When teams know what to do and how to do it, not just by observation but by actually doing it, optimal conditions for success are created.

- Give reminders prior to the assessment: Reminders are helpful! Send reminders to teams with information about what to bring, parking, and anything else they might need to know so they can ensure they're prepared for the assessment.
- Support early arrivals: One of the worst things for teams is to feel late or rushed for an assessment. Evaluators should encourage teams to arrive early. This gives them time to find the location, allow their dog to eliminate in an approved area, and walk around with their dog to become familiar with the setting. Make sure to provide directions on when they can enter the assessment area and instructions around avoiding other teams, who may also be waiting.
- Encourage teams throughout the assessment: Evaluators can be so overly focused on what a team is doing wrong that they forget to share what teams are doing right. Evaluators can encourage teams by stating specific behavioral skills that they did well. For example, and evaluator might say, "I saw how Manny sat the first time you gave a cue. Great job!" This encouragement goes a long way in helping teams feel at ease and, when done at the beginning of the assessment process, helps build confidence in the team.
- Adapt to the presence of volunteers: Teams can be overwhelmed by having several people staring at them; however, teams should be comfortable being in places with other people. Evaluators can direct volunteers to talk quietly with one another, just as if they were people sitting in the hall at a facility. This takes some focus off the team and also presents a more realistic environment reflective of the actual volunteer experience.

Setting up the room, having diverse and well-trained volunteers and making efforts to reduce handler and team stress all contribute to an enjoyable and efficient assessment process.

What to Bring

Preparation for the CAI team assessment is key. Handlers should make sure to bring or turn in all required paperwork, equipment, and resources that are required for team assessment. The paperwork that is typically required includes a handler application or questionnaire, evidence of handler training (if required), and a canine health screening form including a current rabies vaccination certificate. We recommend that CAI organizations make use of an online portal through which teams can upload documents prior to scheduling a team assessment. This way, they can verify that their required documentation has been submitted prior to the assessment day.

As animal behavior organizations increasingly advocate for the use of positive reinforcement training (e.g., IAABC, 2018), CAI organizations have correspondingly clarified their requirements for approved and restricted equipment. The most common approved and restricted equipment or resources for assessments, based on the three CAI organizations previously discussed earlier in this chapter, includes the following:

Approved Equipment/Resources

- collars/harnesses: buckle or snap-in collars in leather, fabric, or synthetic materials; harnesses made of leather or fabric that don't restrict the dog's mobility
- leashes: 6-foot leash or shorter, with some organizations requiring a 4-foot leash
- brushes with soft bristles
- one treat for the *accepting a treat* skill

Restricted Equipment/Resources

- collars/harnesses: pinch, choke, prong, or electronic collars; collars with any metal links; head halters (for some organizations); and harnesses that restrict movement
- leashes: leashes longer than 6 feet, retractable leashes, leashes with a metal chain, and hands-free leashes
- wire bristle brushes or combs with metallic teeth
- any other treats, treat bags, food, toys, and reinforcement tools

Appearance and Grooming

Both handlers and dogs should be groomed and have a professional appearance. Volunteers represent CAI organizations and thus should give a professional impression to facility staff, volunteer coordinators, and CAI clients.

Handler Appearance and Grooming

Handlers should be clean, well groomed, and healthy and not be under the influence of drugs or alcohol. Approved handler attire includes pants, slacks, or capris, business-professional shirts or polos, and shoes with closed toes and straps around the heal. Restricted handler attire includes tight-fitting clothes, short shorts, tank tops, flip flops, high heels, and shoes without backs.

Dog Appearance and Grooming

It's important for dogs to be clean and well groomed for the team assessment and for CAI visits or sessions. Dogs should have trimmed or filed nails and clean teeth, be free of internal and external parasites, and be in overall good general health. Recall our discussion of canine and client welfare covered in Chapter 4.

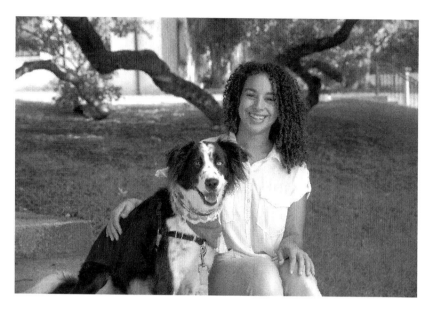

Figure 7.4 CAC team Morgan Rupe and therapy dog Rio are ready to work with clients.

CAI Team Assessment Skills

In this section we'll present CAI team assessment skills. In Chapter 5 we presented the purpose of these skills and why they should be included in both an organization's training and assessment protocols. We'll now describe how to present the skill in a team assessment. The skills in this section were informed and inspired by the skills identified in the assessments used by TDI (2019), Pet Partners (2016), and ATD (2017, 2019). Readers will find new skills here that we believe should be included in CAI team assessments, with a particular focus on handler skills that are often overlooked or, at the very least, underassessed.

Fredrickson and Howie (2000) argued that four criteria should be in place to address the majority of liability concerns across varied CAI settings: (1) reliability, (2) predictability, (3) controllability, and (4) suitability. Our goal is to present CAI team assessment skills that meet these four criteria. The skills that we propose are grouped thematically and are sequentially presented to facilitate the assessment process from the arrival to the departure of the team. The categories of skills include handler check-ins, initial interactions, basic obedience, handling and grooming, walking, crowds, distractions, reaction to a neutral dog, interactions with clients/patients, stay and come when called, setting limits, and accepting and avoiding reinforcers.

Handler Check-In

This skill is typically one of the first skills in the team assessment. Teams are asked to check in and complete paperwork if needed, just as if they were checking in to a new facility with their dog.

 ### Skill 1: Handler Check-In

Skill purpose: To check in with handler, assess handler and canine appearance, and review or verify paperwork.

Skill description: The evaluator greets the handler verbally, without shaking the handler's hand, and reviews paperwork. The evaluator ensures that the handler is dressed appropriately and the dog is wearing an approved collar and leash. The evaluator provides a brief overview of how the evaluator will introduce each skill. The evaluator encourages the handler to talk to and advocate for the dog throughout the team evaluation and ask the evaluator questions, as needed.

Initial Interactions

The initial interaction skills assessed in a team assessment involve how the dog responds to a stranger (i.e., the evaluator) greeting the handler and to being pet by a stranger. Because therapy dogs are often in settings where they are around strangers, it's important for CAI teams to be willing to meet and be comfortable around strangers. What follows is a description of this skill.

 ### Skill 2: Accepting a Friendly Stranger

Skill purpose: To greet handler, assess handler temperament and social skills, and assess the dog's reaction to a stranger shaking hands with the handler.

Skill description: The evaluator approaches the handler and shakes the handler's hand. The evaluator asks the handler to introduce her or his dog. The evaluator also asks, "Why would you like to volunteer with your dog?" The evaluator listens to the handler's responses while observing the dog's behavior.

The second component of Skill 2 sees the evaluator assess how a dog responds to the being pet by a stranger. What follows is a description of this skill.

> **Accepting petting** The evaluator asks the handler if the evaluator can pet the dog. The evaluator then bends down to pet the dog. The dog should welcome the interaction, without backing away or showing signs of aggression.

Related to this skill and as discussed in Chapter 5, assessing how the handler *teaches* a person to greet their dog is important. Recall that when CAI sessions are held in public settings, there may be individuals who have limited experience with dogs and who will require instruction on how to interact with a therapy dog. Here is a description of this skill.

 ### Skill 3: Teaching How to Greet a Dog

Skill purpose: To assess the handler's ability to teach a person how to greet a dog, assess the handler's ability to advocate for the dog, and assess the dog's interest in interacting with a stranger.

Skill description: The evaluator asks the handler if the evaluator can pet the dog. The handler responds that she or he will teach the evaluator how to greet the dog. The handler then asks the evaluator to approach the dog slowly from the side, stand still (or kneel down and stay still, if the handler has a small dog), and allow the dog to approach and smell the evaluator. When the dog has finished smelling the evaluator, then the handler instructs the evaluator to rub the dog on the chest, back, or other places where the dog likes to be pet. If needed, the handler should indicate places where the dog doesn't like to be pet (e.g., "My dog doesn't like being pet on the head or tail, but she really likes getting chest scratches or belly rubs.").

By assessing this skill as part of the team assessment, CAI organizations can evaluate how handlers facilitate dog greetings with strangers and set limits for interactions, especially for people with limited experience interacting with dogs, as well as how the dog responds to accepting petting.

Basic Obedience, Handling, and Grooming

Basic obedience skills, handling, and grooming are essential for CAI teams. Therapy dogs should be able to demonstrate sit, down, stay, and come when called. We present each of these skills in turn.

Skill 4: Sit

Skill purpose: To evaluate how the dog responds to the handler's cue to sit.

Skill description: The evaluator asks the handler to cue the dog to sit. The handler cues the dog to sit. The evaluator then assesses the delivery of the cue by the handler and compliance to the cue by the dog.

 ## Skill 5: Handling

Skill purpose: To assess the dog's overall health and response to being handled.

Skill description: While the dog is in a sitting position, the evaluator looks at the dog's eyes and in the dog's ears and checks all four paws and the dog's nails.

 ## Skill 6: Down

Skill purpose: To evaluate how the dog responds to the handler's cue to down.

Skill description: The evaluator asks the handler to cue the dog to a down position. The handler cues the dog to down. The evaluator then assesses the handler's delivery of the cue and the dog's compliance.

 ## Skill 7: Grooming

Skill purpose: To assess the dog's appearance and grooming.

Skill description: While the dog is in a down position, the evaluator assesses the dog's appearance by petting the dog's body and tail. The evaluator then takes a soft-bristle brush and brushes the dog's fur three times. The evaluator assesses the handler's interaction and dog's reaction during this skill.

Walking Skills

A therapy dog should be able to walk calmly by the handler's side and demonstrate to people in the facility that both the handler and dog are walking and working well together. As mentioned in Chapter 5, the evaluator is looking for the leash to be loose between the handler and dog, where the leash drops down and looks like a J-shape between the handler and dog. The evaluator is also looking to see that the dog is able to walk calmly next to the handler when the handler turns in different directions and when the handler stops. This demonstrates that the dog is focused on the handler and will allow the handler to lead in both relaxed and stressful situations.

 ### Skill 8: Walking on a Loose Leash

Skill purpose: To assess how the handler and dog walk together and to ensure the dog can walk calmly next to the handler with a loose leash.

Skill description: *An L-shape that is 10 feet straight ahead and 10 feet to the right will be taped on the floor prior to the evaluation.* The evaluator will ask the team to walk on the L-shaped line, making turns as indicated, and turn and walk back when they get to the end of the line. Before the teams starts, the evaluator instructs the team that he or she will stop the team at some point while they are walking. The evaluator will stop the team just after they get to the end of the L, turn around, and start walking back.

Crowd Skills

CAI handlers and therapy dogs should be prepared for walking in crowds and having several people approach the dog at once. Evaluating how the handler and the dog manage crowds is important for assessing the team's ability to withstand stressors. We believe that all CAI organizations should evaluate how handlers and dogs walk in crowds and manage several people wanting to pet the dog as this reflects strong ecological validity—teams are likely to encounter this in their role as volunteers or practitioners. Assessment volunteers who participate in this skill should reflect the diversity of people in the community and in the CAI context in which the team will most likely be working.

 ### Skill 9: Walking Through a Crowd

Skill purpose: To assess how teams manage walking through a crowd.

Skill description: The evaluator will ask the team to walk in a straight line toward the back of the room. While the team is walking, a person walking unsteadily with a walker, crutches, or mobility aid will walk in front of the team from the left; another person (walking steadily) will walk in front of the team from the right; and a third person will walk behind the team from the right.

As discussed in Chapter 5, we believe that it's important for handlers to be able to manage and set limits with people who want to pet the dog. Handlers have the right and responsibility to decide how many people can pet their dog at the same time, how the dog is positioned, and how the interactions take place. The assessment should include a child volunteer and a volunteer using a wheelchair to evaluate how teams respond to children and assistive equipment. Here is the description for this skill.

Skill 10: Managing Several People Who Want to Pet the Dog

Skill purpose: To assess how the handler manages several people who want to pet the dog at the same time.

Skill description: The evaluator tells the handler that the three people approaching want to pet the dog, one of whom is a child and another of whom is in a wheelchair. The handler instructs all three people to space out next to each other, about a foot apart. The handler states that each person will take a turn petting the dog. The handler teaches all three people how to greet the dog (as presented in the *teaching how to greet a dog* skill). The handler then allows the dog to sniff and greet each person. The handler will bring the dog next to the person in the wheelchair or pick the dog up, if the dog is a small dog.

Facilitating the skill this way allows the handler to demonstrate assertiveness, their ability to manage and set limits for approaching clients to prevent their dog from being overcrowded, and their ability to safeguard canine welfare.

Distraction Skills

The purpose of assessing how CAI teams react to distractions is to see how each member of the team responds during unexpected instances or events. All three of the assessments we propose in the sections that follow assess distraction skills. We chose distractions that would be most commonly found in facilities: a person jogging by (e.g., a doctor, nurse, or child getting to another destination) and the sound of a vacuum. Here is the description of this skill.

 ### Skill 11: Reaction to Distractions

Skill purpose: To assess how the team responds to distractions while walking.

    Skill description: The evaluator will ask the team to walk in a straight line toward the front of the room. While the team is walking, a person will jog by in front of the team from the left and a person in the back of the room will turn on a vacuum for three seconds (this sound should be consistent across all team assessments).

Reactions to a Team With a Neutral Dog

As more and more helping dogs are introduced into public settings, it's essential that therapy dogs are assessed for their reaction to a neutral dog, such as a service dog. As our goal is to comprehensively assess CAI teams and ensure teams are suitable for public work, we hold that therapy dogs should be able to pass by, and be near, another team without reacting or interacting with a neutral dog. The skill is described next.

 ### Skill 12: Reaction to a Team With a Neutral Dog

Skill purpose: To assess how the team responds to a neutral dog.

    Skill description: The evaluator will ask the team to walk to the opposite end of the room and invite a neutral dog team to enter the room. Both dogs should be placed on the outside (e.g., if a dog walks on the left side of the handler, both dogs would walk on the left side of their handlers and the handlers would walk toward each other, so the handlers are passing each other). The evaluator asks both teams to walk toward each other and directs the handlers to stop next to each other, shake hands, and briefly greet each other. The dog in the team being assessed should not cross in front of the handler to interact with either member of the neutral dog team when the handlers pause to greet each other. The evaluator will direct both teams to continue walking after the brief greeting. The neutral dog team should leave the room immediately after this skill is completed.

Stay and Come When Called

These basic obedience skills are important for CAI teams in settings in which the dog may need to *stay* in a certain place for safety reasons or so the handler can talk to another person. Similarly, *come when called* may be important if the dog finds interest in a person, other animal, or object with which the dog shouldn't be interacting. We recognize that therapy dogs in volunteer settings should be on a leash; nevertheless, this skill is important as it reflects the handler's ability to direct the dog and it reflects too the handler/dog relationship. These two skills can be assessed one right after the other.

 Skill 13: Stay

Skill purpose: To assess how the dog responds to the handler's cue to stay.

Skill description: The evaluator asks the handler to hold onto the leash, attach the long leash, then hold onto the long leash, and take the original leash off. This process ensures that the dog is on leash at all times. The evaluator asks the handler to cue the dog to a sit or down position, and then cue the dog to stay. The evaluator then asks the handler to face away from the dog, walk 10 feet away, then turn around and face the dog. The evaluator then asks the handler to pause for 3 seconds, then walk back to the dog.

 Skill 14: Come When Called

Skill purpose: To assess how the dog responds to the handler's cue to come when called.

Skill description: The dog should stay in a sit or down position from the previous skill. The evaluator asks the handler to cue the dog to stay. The evaluator then asks the handler to face away from the dog, walk 10 feet away, then turn around and face the dog. The evaluator then asks the handler to pause for 3 seconds, then cue the dog to come.

Setting Limits

In Chapter 5 we presented a model for setting limits called the ACT model, developed by Landreth (2012). To recap, the model has three steps:

- A: Acknowledge the person's wishes or wants.
- C: Communicate the limit.
- T: Target an alternate behavior.

This skill is especially important when teams work with unpredictable clients. Here are two skills that allow handlers to demonstrate their limit-setting skills.

 Skill 15: Setting a Limit – Restraining Hug

Skill purpose: To assess how the handler sets limits with a person who wants to hug the dog.

Skill description: The evaluator and handler sit down on the floor with the dog. The evaluator tells the handler that she or he is going to pretend to start the hug the dog and that the handler needs to interrupt and demonstrate the ACT model to set a limit with the evaluator. The evaluator then states, "I'd really like to hug your dog" and starts to reach for the dog to hug the dog. The handler should put her or his hand out to prevent the evaluator from hugging the dog and use the ACT wording to set limits with the evaluator (e.g., "I can see that you'd like to hug my dog, but my dog is not for hugging like that. She prefers to be pet on the chest or get belly rubs.").

 Skill 16: Setting a Limit – Request to Take Dog

Skill purpose: To assess how the handler sets limits with a person who wants to take the dog with him or her and away from the handler.

Skill description: The evaluator tells the handler that she or he is going to pretend to be a volunteer coordinator who would like to take the dog to meet some staff members in a staff-only area. The evaluator tells the handler to demonstrate the ACT model with this request. The evaluator then states, "Could I take your dog with me really quick to meet the staff?" and starts to reach for the dog's leash. The handler should put her or his hand out to prevent the evaluator from taking the leash and use the ACT wording to set limits with the evaluator (e.g., "I can tell that you'd like to take my dog with you to meet the staff, but my dog has to stay with me at all times because we're a team. My dog and I can come with you into the staff area, or you can bring the staff out here to meet us.").

Accepting and Avoiding Reinforcers

The cue *leave it* is often used to teach dogs when to leave an item alone, such as a toy, medication, or food. In varied CAI settings, therapy dogs may find food or medication lying on the floor. Therapy dogs responding consistently to this skill is important, as ingesting medication can be dangerous.

Skill 17: Leave It

Skill purpose: To assess how the dog responds when the dog is presented with an opportunity to eat something on the floor and is not allowed to eat it.

Skill description: The evaluator asks the team to walk past a bowl with a treat in it on the ground. The handler can cue the dog to "leave it" once. The dog is not allowed to lick or eat the treat.

Giving treats can be beneficial in establishing, building, and enhancing a therapy dog's relationship with clients. We argue that this skill should be optional and that handlers can determine whether they want to allow strangers to feed their dog treats. As dogs are typically joyful when receiving treats, this is a positive way to end a CAI team assessment.

 Skill 18: Accepting a Treat

Skill purpose: To assess how the handler guides a person in offering a treat and to assess how the dog responds to accepting a treat.

Skill description: The evaluator asks the handler if she or he can give the dog a treat. The handler instructs the evaluator on how to give a treat (e.g., "To give my dog a treat, make your hand flat or cupped like this and put your fingers together. Then put a treat in center of your hand and ask the dog to sit. When the dog is sitting, lower your hand under the dog's mouth so the dog can take the treat."). The dog should gently take the treat from the evaluator's hand.

Reviewing Assessment Outcomes and Next Steps

CAI team evaluators should be sufficiently trained and assessed in facilitating an assessment prior to conducting one. For each skill, evaluators should use behavioral criteria that clearly describes how the handler and dog are to behave during the interaction. Examples of behavioral criteria are provided in the following rubric. Both handlers and dogs should be scored for each skill. There are three outcome categories for behavioral responses: *pass, not ready,* or *unsuitable*. Evaluators should check each of the behavioral responses that a handler or dog meets or demonstrates as part of a skill assessment. For example, if a handler provides clear directions, facilitates the interaction, and responds to canine stress signals, then the evaluator would check *all* three behavioral responses. Evaluators should select all behavioral responses, even if the responses are found in different categories. For example, if a dog showed positive canine signals, such as having an open mouth and relaxed posture, but needed three cues from the handler to come when called, the evaluator should check "Displays positive canine signals" and "Responds to handler's cues after two or more cues." In addition to checking each behavioral response, evaluators should include written examples of a handler or dog's response. An example of this is "Gave clear directions on how to give a treat" for the handler and "Took treat gently" for the dog. Evaluators can and should pause between each skill to write such brief notes.

The skill rating corresponds to the three outcome categories found on the rubric: pass, not ready, and unsuitable. The skill rating should be given for each skill in the assessment, and for both the handler and dog. Sometimes handlers or dogs may demonstrate behaviors from different skills categories, such as behaviors from the pass category and the unsuitable category. If a handler or dog demonstrates even one behavioral response that is checked in a category other than pass, the skill rating should be for the category of the lowest behavioral response. For example, if a dog responds to a handler's first cue to sit (e.g., in the pass category) but then growls and lunges at the evaluator (e.g., in the unsuitable category), then the skill rating is unsuitable.

If the handler and dog both earn a pass rating in all skills in the assessment, then the team passes the assessment and can move forward with CAI team credentialing. Teams who earn a not ready rating on certain skills and do not receive any unsuitable ratings should practice the skills in which they struggled and then reevaluate when the team is able to demonstrate the skill meeting expectations and the CAI organization has another assessment day scheduled. If a handler or dog earns an unsuitable rating on any skill, then the handler or dog are not an ideal fit for work in CAI and should debrief with the evaluator.

CAI Team Assessment Scoring

Handler	Dog
Pass:	**Pass:**
○ Provides clear directions on how a person should approach and interact with the dog. ○ Touches, talks to, and assesses the dog while another person is interacting with the dog and throughout each skill.	○ Responds to handler's cues after the first cue. ○ Seeks out interactions with the evaluation volunteers, including the evaluator.

Handler	Dog
o Clearly describes where the dog likes and doesn't like to be pet. o Facilitates the interaction by talking to both the dog and person while the person is interacting the dog. o Responds to any canine stress signals immediately.	o Displays positive canine signals. o Displays minimal canine stress signals but recovers quickly.

Not ready:

o Does not provide clear directions on how to approach and interact with the dog. o Does not touch, talk to, or assess the dog while another person is interacting with the dog. o Does not facilitate the interaction. o Is overly anxious or lacks social skills. o Responds to canine stress signals late.	o Responds to handler's cues after two or more cues. o Backs away or is hesitant around the evaluator or evaluation volunteers. o Jumps on, barks at, or excessively licks the evaluator or evaluation volunteers. o Displays minimal canine stress signals but doesn't recover quickly.

Unsuitable:

o Does not provide any directions on how to interact with the dog. o Forces the dog to do something that the dog doesn't want to do. o Doesn't respond to canine stress signals.	o Does not respond to handler's cues. o Displays significant stress signals. o Growls or shows aggressive behavior toward any person or animal before, during, or after the evaluation.

Notes:

Handler skill rating:

☐ Pass
☐ Not ready
☐ Unsuitable

Notes:

Dog skill rating:

☐ Pass
☐ Not ready
☐ Unsuitable

Knowing how to effectively review feedback with teams is an important skill for evaluators. One of the best ways to start assessment feedback is to ask the handler to share what they thought about how the assessment went. If a team has struggled with some skills in the assessment, it's helpful for the *handler* to talk about these things first. The evaluator can encourage this by asking the handler, "What are two skills you thought went well and what are two skills with which you or your dog struggled?" It is much easier to discuss areas of growth if the handler can acknowledge the areas of growth first.

After asking about the handler's initial thoughts regarding the assessment, the evaluator should review each skill and discuss the behavioral responses checked and any notes. The evaluator should emphasize what the team did well. For assessments in which the team earned a pass for all skills, the evaluator should acknowledge their competence and discuss next steps in the credentialing process.

For *not ready* skill ratings, the evaluator should share with the handler what they observed and what the handler or dog should do differently in the future. For example, if the dog required three cues to sit, the evaluator could share with the handler, "When you come for the assessment next time, your dog needs to be able to sit after the first cue that you give." If there is an opportunity for the evaluator to demonstrate the skill, this could be helpful. For example, if a handler has not practiced teaching a person how to greet a dog or how to use the ACT limit-setting model, the evaluator could briefly show the team how to do this or provide resources, such as a link to an online video demonstrating these skills. The evaluator can ask the handler what the handler thinks could help them work on areas of growth. The evaluator could also offer the handler referrals for positive reinforcement trainers who understand the skills that are assessed in the CAI assessment. Finally, it's helpful for evaluators to check in with handlers at the end of the feedback discussion. Some handlers go into assessments believing that they will pass the first time and that CAI assessments are a relatively easy process. If handlers don't pass the first time, they may be disappointed or concerned that they were not meant to be a CAI team. Evaluators should be prepared to support handlers in acknowledging strengths, areas for growth, and how to move forward.

For teams who receive an *unsuitable* rating for any skill, it's important for evaluators to emphasize that CAI work should be a fit for both the handler and the dog. We also want dogs to enjoy, and not just tolerate, CAI with others. Think of situations in your own life in which you felt extremely stressed or miserable because you had to tolerate something. Volunteering as a CAI team should be something where both the handler and dog are both suitable for CAI work and derive enjoyment from it. The evaluator should discuss other options with the handler. This could include, depending on who received the unsuitable rating, partnering with a different dog, partnering with another person's dog (with permission), working with another animal species, such as a rabbit or guinea pig, and volunteering at a facility without a dog. These options all provide opportunities to help and support people, which is the primary goal of CAI. It's important, too, for CAI team evaluators to be reflective and, should they see a high number of teams fail, to successfully navigate their assessment protocol, reflection on the training provided to teams must be undertaken. Some questions for reflection are:

- Were teams sufficiently trained and prepared for the assessment?
- Did the evaluator focus more on what the team didn't do well?
- How can the CAI organization or evaluator help to better prepare teams in the future?

Conclusion

This chapter examined the elements of the CAI team assessment. We explored why assessment is important and the purpose for, and challenges in, assessing CAI teams. We provided an overview of CAI team assessments from three different CAI organizations. We also discussed how to set up and prepare for CAI team assessments. Next, building on the foundation provided in Chapter 5, we provided a description of each skill requiring assessment, including how to score and determine credentialing outcomes for teams. In our next chapter we'll examine assessment considerations for teams working in specialized contexts.

References

Alliance of Therapy Dogs (ATD). (2017). *ATD test demo*. Retrieved January 5, 2019, from https://vimeo.com/184999407

Alliance of Therapy Dogs (ATD). (2019). *ATD information packet*. Retrieved January 5, 2019, from https://j3uv01gyifh3iqdfjuwz0qip-wpengine.netdna-ssl.com/wp-content/uploads/2018/12/2019-Info-Pkt-pdf.pdf

American Kennel Club (AKC). (2018). *What is Canine Good Citizen?* Retrieved December 30, 2018, from www.akc.org/products-services/training-programs/canine-good-citizen/what-is-canine-good-citizen/

Binfet, J., & Struik, K. (2018). Dogs on campus. *Society & Animals*, early online edition. doi: 10.1163/15685306–12341495.

Butler, K. (2013). *Therapy dogs today: Their gifts, our obligation* (2nd ed.). Norman, OK: Funpuddle Publishing Associates.

Fredrickson, M., & Howie, A. R. (2000). Methods, standards, guidelines, and considerations in selecting animals for animal-assisted therapy: Part B: Guidelines and standards for animal selection in animal-assisted activity and therapy programs. In A. H. Fine (Ed.), *Handbook on animal-assisted therapy: Theoretical foundations and guidelines for practice* (pp. 99–114). San Diego, CA: Academic Press.

Fredrickson-MacNamara, M., & Butler, K. (2010). Animal selection procedures in animal-assisted interaction programs. In A. H. Fine (Ed.), *Handbook on animal-assisted therapy* (3rd ed., pp. 111–134). Amsterdam: Elsevier.

International Association of Animal Behavior Consultants (IAABC). (2018). *Hierarchy of procedures for humane and effective practice*. Retrieved from https://m.iaabc.org/about/position-statements/lima/hierarchy/

Jones, A. C., & Gosling, S. D. (2005). Temperament and personality in dogs (canis familiaris): A review and evaluation of past research. *Applied Animal Behaviour Science*, 95, 1–53. doi: 10.1016/j.applanim.2005.04.008.

Landreth, G. (2012). *Play therapy: The art of the relationship* (3rd ed.). New York: Brunner Routledge.

Pet Partners. (2016). *Pet Partners team evaluation: Skills exercises for dogs.* Retrieved January 5, 2019, from https://petpartners.org/wp-content/uploads/2015/06/Evaluation Overview_Dogs.pdf

Pet Partners. (2019). *About us.* Retrieved January 7, 2019, from https://petpartners.org/about-us/

Taylor, K. D., & Mills, D. S. (2006). The development and assessment of temperament tests for adult companion dogs. *Journal of Veterinary Behavior: Clinical Applications and Research, 1,* 94–108. doi: 10.1016/j.jveb.2006.09.002.

Therapy Dogs International (TDI). (2019). *For the record.* Retrieved January 5, 2019, from www.tdi-dog.org/default.aspx

8 Assessment Considerations for Specialized Contexts

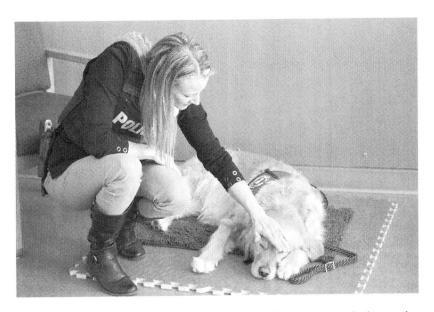

Figure 8.1 A Royal Canadian Mounted Police constable interacts with therapy dog Dash at the City of Kelowna Detachment.

This chapter builds upon the foundation we established in Chapter 5, which outlined the basic training a prospective CAI team should undergo in preparation for assessment leading to credentialing. The aim of this chapter is to provide an overview for readers of settings and client profiles for which the CAI team requires additional, more extensive training and assessment in order to optimally support client well-being. We will begin by defining a specialized context, provide arguments for why additional training for CAI teams is warranted within these contexts, and then provide illustrations of the additional training required for work in varied specialized environments including educational, law enforcement, health care, airport, and crisis response settings. Our aim here is not to highlight the benefits of CAIs within each of these contexts, recognizing that for some of these contexts there is not yet corresponding empirical evidence to support CAIs within these settings, but rather to present to readers the complexities of CAI teams working in varied, nuanced environments and to provoke thinking around placing CAI teams in novel settings.

Scenario

As a long-time dog enthusiast in her town, Susan is the founder and director of a small CAI organization that brings dogs to a local retirement facility to support seniors. She has a reliable team of 15 dogs in any given year who help with this. Susan does her own assessments of dogs, and this model has worked well for the last 10 years. She never has trouble finding volunteer dog handlers, and many relatives of the senior residents of the facility end up volunteering. Occasionally, Susan will agree to a school visit or presentation to showcase the work her organization is doing, and they have received good press for their work in the community, having been on the news over the years and in the local paper several times. A new principal at the local elementary school approached Susan about having therapy dogs come into the school to help reluctant readers. The principal received a grant and some of the funds could help buy vests for the dogs in Susan's program. She's tempted but this forges new ground for her and her dog/handler teams. Susan wonders about the intricacies of having dogs in a school and if her dog/handler teams are up for this task.

Questions for Reflection and Discussion

1. Would a dog who is good with seniors automatically be good with children?
2. Would the handlers have to receive training around how to teach reading?
3. What if a child misbehaves? Whose responsibility is it to manage that?

What Is a Specialized Context?

As we outlined in our first chapter, the field of CAI has grown and has moved beyond the stereotypic image of a therapy dog visiting a senior in a retirement home. As we've illustrated throughout this book, we now see therapy dogs working in a variety of specialized contexts. For the purposes of this chapter, a specialized context is a context in which advanced training by the therapy dog and/or the handler is required in order for CAIs to be successful. The context might be rendered "specialized" because of any or all of the following:

- The setting is high in stimuli (this might include a high volume of clients and/or a busy, public setting).

- The client population supported by the CAI team is complex (this might include clients with acute stress or clients with challenging mental or physical health) and the resultant demand on the CAI team is high.
- There is a high level of unpredictability characterizing the setting (no two visits to this setting are the same for the CAI team given ever-changing clients or movement by the CAI team within the setting).

As a general rule or guideline, we might rank the contexts in which CAI teams work on a continuum of low to high environmental stimuli, low to high demand on the CAI team pending the client profile they are supporting, and low to high unpredictability. A low-stimuli and low-demand context might see a CAI team support one client in a static setting. The demand on the CAI team is relatively low with the session composed of interactions between the three agents—therapy dog, handler, and client. The setting is relatively quiet, with little external stimuli and with little foot traffic in an out of the setting. The routine for the dog and handler is familiar, and there is little unpredictability in what unfolds during a session. The CAI team is working independent of other CAI teams, and the setting might be characterized by little noise. In short, there are few distractions. The demand of the handler is largely conversational, and a rapport may have been established with the client over time. The tasks required of the handler are familiar and the demand of the handler can be considered low.

A high-demand or high-stimuli environment could be considered a setting in which the CAI team addresses any or all of the following (see Table 8.1):

Table 8.1 Criteria Defining a Specialized Context for Canine-Assisted Interventions

Environmental Considerations	*Client Considerations*
A dynamic or public setting in which the CAI team is mobile	High volume or number of clients
Auditory and olfactory distractions present (e.g., overhead announcements, food)	High turnover rate of clients with the unscheduled arrival and departure of clients
Working in proximity to other dogs (i.e., therapy, service, or pet) or animals	Cultural and ethnic diversity in the clients interacting with the dog
Exposure to objects with wheels (e.g., suitcases, strollers, wheelchairs, etc.)	Diversity in the ages of clients (e.g., children to senior citizens)
Working in environments with specialized equipment (e.g., health-related machinery)	Clients with negative or few experiences with dogs
A setting in which employees are performing routine tasks concurrent with canine visit	Clients with amplified and complex emotional states (e.g., stress, anxious, upset)
	Clients with complex physical health profiles

The Importance of CAI Team Training for Specialized Settings

As we have highlighted throughout this book, there is variability in how CAI teams are screened, assessed, and trained for participation in CAIs. Across all of the different CAI organizations in operation, we see a wide array of screening, assessment, and training practices used, and this has been reported in our own research (Hartwig & Binfet, 2019) and in recent research by others (e.g., Linder, Siebens, Mueller, Gibbs, & Freeman, 2017). Correspondingly, we also see substandard screening and assessment practices used by organizations to identify the fitness of CAI teams for work in CAIs (e.g., using only the Canine Good Citizen test). The danger of inadequate screening, training, and assessment practices places all stakeholders at risk and puts the public in an especially precarious position as they may encounter dogs who are ill-suited to participating in CAIs. Related to the inadequate screening, training, and assessment of therapy dogs is the inadequate screening and training of handlers for work in specialized contexts. This is especially important when handlers are asked to work in complex environments and support clients with complex needs or behavioral profiles. In light of the popularity and growth of CAIs, we argue here that CAI teams working in specialized contexts must undergo additional and nuanced assessment and training. In the sections that follow, we review some of these specialized contexts.

Illustrations of Specialized Contexts

What follows next are illustrations of training and assessment considerations for CAI teams working in specialized contexts. The contexts we've chosen to illustrate are by no means an exhaustive list of the specialized contexts in which CAI teams might be asked to work and for which they require specialized training. The curated examples here are presented to illustrate and reinforce the notion that the standard credential of "therapy dog" does not sufficiently prepare the CAI team for work within these contexts. It is our intention here to raise awareness around the additional training and assessment considerations for CAI teams participating in CAIs taking place in specialized contexts so they may optimally support client well-being.

Educational Contexts

Public Schools

A popular reason we might see therapy dogs in schools is for canine-assisted reading programs (Fung, 2017; Hall, Gee, & Mills, 2016; Lane & Zavada, 2013, Le Roux, Swartz, & Swart, 2014). Therapy dogs within this context are sometimes referred to as "reading dogs," and along with their handlers, they help create a nonthreatening context within which young students can practice their oral reading skills. Struggling readers are encouraged to read aloud to a therapy dog as a way of strengthening their reading skills and reading confidence. Obviously, therapy dogs working in this context must be assessed for compatibility with children, and handlers must have a current criminal record background check completed in order for the CAI team to work in this context. In light of all of the paper and paper products in this setting, there is an increased risk that dogs in a school context could step on a dropped staple and, as is standard practice, the room should be cleaned and prepped for the dog's visit. Therapy dogs working in reading programs need to be especially calm, as they typically sit or lie next to the child and play a relatively placid interactive role. The dog cannot be seeking attention from the child by pawing at the child and must be able to settle quickly and remain settled for the duration of the session. Therapy dogs in this context work under the direct supervision of their handler, and handlers are cognizant they are not teachers within this context and should be prepared to follow program guidelines around helping children focus, responding to children's questions, encouraging positive behaviors, and redirecting off-task behaviors. Handlers working in school reading programs should be trained in reporting suspected neglect and abuse or the disclosure of neglect or abuse by a child and understand their role as a public guardian of child welfare. A handler who suspects neglect or abuse or is the recipient of disclosed information of neglect or abuse by a child is required to follow CAI organization and school policies and report suspected abuse or neglect to the local child protection agency (e.g., Child Protective Services in the United States).

College Campuses

In scanning research investigating the effects of CAIs, the postsecondary or college campus setting is a popular setting in which to investigate the effects on well-being of spending time with therapy dogs. This is perhaps not surprising as there is keen interest on the part of college-age students to spend time with dogs, and there are ample professionals within this context who are equipped to carry out studies that, in turn, are published. Specifically, researchers are curious to explore the effect that spending time with therapy dogs has on student stress reduction, anxiety, and homesickness. Though the methodologies vary somewhat, across campuses and researchers, we see several studies reporting the positive effects of spending time with therapy dogs (e.g., Barker, Barker, McCain, & Schubert, 2016; Crossman, Kazdin, & Knudson, 2015; Pendry & Vandagriff, 2019; Ward-Griffin et al., 2018).

Therapy dogs working in a postsecondary setting must be especially well screened as they typically work in busy, high-stimulus public spaces and the interest on the part of students to interact with therapy dogs often surpasses the organization's capacity. As with therapy dogs in public schools, the risk of dropped food, medication, and staples is ever present, and the room or space in which dogs are to work must be cleaned and prepped.

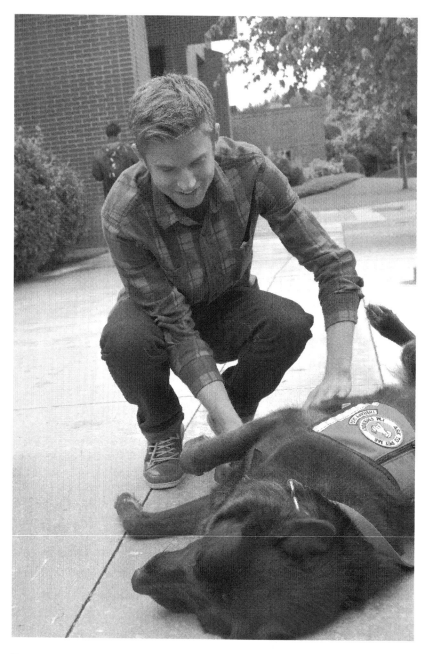

Figure 8.2 A student at the University of British Columbia interacts with therapy dog Siska.

Given the popularity of CAIs on college campuses, handlers working in on-campus stress-reduction programs must be confident in establishing parameters for students attending sessions. This might include reminding students not to pick up dogs, not to roughhouse with dogs, not to feed dogs, and to temper their excitement so as to not overexcite dogs within a session. Handlers must also receive training on how to support students in distress—either observed during their interaction with the dog/handler team or through a self-disclosure by a visiting student. Handlers must thus be aware of signs of distress (e.g., low affect) and aware of the on-campus resources available to students so that students may be redirected to additional sources of support. CAI organization personnel must be informed by handlers of students in distress so that campus personnel can follow up with individual students (recall our discussion of the Question, Persuade, Refer (QPR) training in Chapter 4).

Law Enforcement Contexts

Police Precincts

As a result of studies on college campuses attesting to the stress-reducing benefits of spending time with therapy dogs, there has been an increased interest in having therapy dogs support the well-being of employees in varied contexts (Binfet, Draper, & Green, in press). One such context is the police precinct, where both first-responding officers and precinct staff are known to have elevated levels of occupational stress (Violanti et al., 2018).

Three distinct formats appear to have been piloted thus far. First, and outside the purview of this book given our focus on therapy dogs, is where a precinct welcomes a certified *facility dog* to support employee well-being. Under the supervision of an employee and housed within the precinct during regularly scheduled hours, the thinking here is that providing routine opportunities to interact with a facility dog will lower stress and boost well-being. The second iteration underway is one in which an employee within the precinct who has a credentialed therapy dog brings the dog to work to allow for informal interactions throughout the working day for employees seeking to feel better through CAI. Last, a more formal and structured iteration of CAI within a police precinct sees a team of therapy dogs brought into the precinct to allow opportunities for employees to interact with therapy dogs. This model is similar to the model used on college campuses that might have a "drop-in" session of sorts that does not require registration of signing up in order to participate in a session with the dogs.

Handlers who participate in CAIs within a precinct will be required to undergo advanced security clearance, be escorted into the building by precinct personnel, sign-in and obtain a visitor identification badge, and remain with their dog in the designated area until escorted out of the building. It is recommended that handlers undergo training led by personnel from their CAI organization who work cooperatively and in liaison with officers from the precinct in order to learn about the precinct culture, as well as the needs of the officers who will visit the dog/handler stations. Similar to the protocol used with college students who may share thoughts of self-harm, handlers working with police officers must be trained in the protocol to follow should a client disclose thoughts of self-harm or appear distressed and in need of additional support. Again, personnel within the precinct are to provide training to handlers on the protocol to follow in these situations.

Only seasoned or experienced CAI teams should work in police precincts to support officer well-being. This is not the context for inexperienced CAI teams. The challenges for therapy dogs working in police precincts include:

- remaining calm in the lobby while awaiting their escort into the precinct, as the lobby can be busy with members of the public arriving and leaving;
- becoming familiarized with the uniform worn by officers;
- becoming familiarized with the work-related paraphernalia worn by officers;
- being assessed for their reaction to the smell of firearms; and
- interacting with clients who may be characterized by acute stress.

Health Care Contexts

Hospitals

Within a health care context, we see CAI teams volunteering or participating in research initiatives in hospitals, and the teams working within this setting must undergo additional screening, training, and assessment. In light of the complex setting and client profile, the hospital setting may be considered a specialized context. The setting itself is complex, as it can be busy and there is a variety of novel stimuli to which dogs must adjust, including machinery and motorized mobility aids. In fact, the setting can be rife with distractions as staff go about their routine duties while CAI teams interact with clients. The client profiles found within this setting can also be complex, with clients having compromised health and/or requiring assistance in their interactions with therapy dogs.

Considerations for handlers working in this context include:

- completion of a criminal record background check in order to work with vulnerable populations (e.g., children, elderly);
- not volunteering when handler health is compromised (e.g., has a cold);
- strong observational skills to avoid dog consuming dropped medication/ food; and
- strong perspective-taking and situational awareness, as the CAI team is in a context in which regular work duties must be performed by multiple employees concurrent with dog/handler visit.

Considerations for therapy dogs working in a hospital setting include:

- giving the dog a bath within 24 hours prior to the visit and ensuring the dog is properly groomed;
- following CAI organization policy regarding diet (recall our discussion of this topic in Chapter 4);
- assessing the dog's reaction to novel stimuli found in a hospital (e.g., riding an elevator, motorized mobility devices, flooring); and
- having a strong "leave it" response should dropped medication or food be encountered.

Airports

Certainly, when we review the table at the beginning of this chapter outlining factors determining a low to high stimuli and demand environment, the airport context is an environment in which almost all of the criteria for a complex, high-stimuli and high-demand environment are found. It is perhaps here, more than any other context in which CAI teams find themselves volunteering, that a challenging context and client profiles are presented. The airport context is especially replete with novel stimuli, varied clients, and unforeseen challenges. The popularity of therapy dogs in airports is reflected by Fodor's Travel (2019) website, which maintains a list, albeit incomplete, of airports that provide access to therapy dogs. As we note in Chapter 10, this is

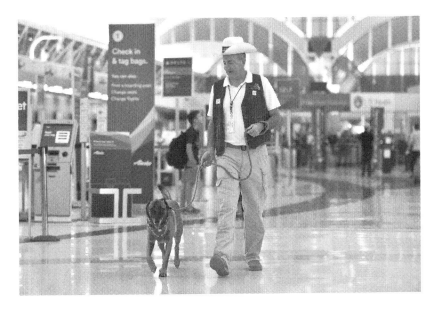

Figure 8.3 A handler and his therapy dog supporting travelers in an airport.

very likely an area of CAIs that will see additional growth with more and more airports partnering with CAI organizations to support traveler well-being.

CAI teams volunteering in this context need to be especially well screened. Given the volume of clients the handler must greet and welcome, the varied ages and diversity of these people, and their likely elevated stress from traveling, handlers need strong social and emotional skills. They also need strong observational skills within this context in order to interact with the public and simultaneously monitor and safeguard their dog's welfare. As part of this volunteer assignment, handlers are encouraged to track the number of visitors they greet within a session. Tracking this helps determine the impact of the session on dogs. What is a reasonable number of clients for an airport dog to greet? The number of clients alone is not entirely indicative of the toll on the airport therapy dog, as clients with elevated stress might be considered high-demand clients and have an exacerbated impact on dogs.

Dogs working in this environment must certainly be assessed for their reaction to children who may break free from a parent's grasp and run toward a nearby or passing dog. Dogs also need to be assessed to gauge their reaction to culturally and ethnically diverse clients. As we discussed in Chapter 3, dogs can have strong reactions to dark skin pigments (Coren, 2016). This assessment would also include assessing the dog's reaction to varied clothing or garb worn by clients. A client wearing an unfamiliar hat or a head covering not previously encountered by the dog can potentially provoke a fear or protective response on the part of the dog.

A further complexity presented by travelers in airports, especially large international airports, is the range of dog knowledge or prior experience clients have. Clients may be drawn to the dog but fearful given the role dogs hold in their respective culture or they may have an unorthodox interaction style that might see them pat the dog on the head rather than gently stroking the dog in a downward motion. It is here that a skilled handler can help navigate such interactions. In light of the number of clients seen by a CAI team in an airport, opportunities for handwashing or disinfecting hands for both the handler and the clients who interact with dogs must be provided.

Crisis Response

Public Tragedies

Therapy dogs are increasingly seen at the site of public tragedies (e.g., mass shootings, floods, fires; USA TODAY, 2018). Therapy dogs working within this context are often referred to as "comfort dogs" (Seattle Times, 2017). Understandably, the CAI team working to provide comfort to victims and mourners after a public tragedy could be described as working in intensified conditions vis-à-vis typical CAI teams.

First, unless the team is local, the dog and handler would be required, on a moment's notice, to travel to the site of the tragedy. Therapy dogs must thus be accustomed to travel and not be distressed by travel. Second, we made a case in our chapter on canine welfare that therapy dogs must be allowed to become familiar with their working environment, and as cited Serpell and colleagues (2010, p. 483), "Animals need to have an opportunity to habituate to the environment and to the activities in which they are involved." Adding a layer of complexity to therapy dogs working to support mourners and victims after a public tragedy is that the CAI team may work in multiple locations (e.g., at an outdoor park near the site of the tragedy to support the public and in hospital rooms to support individual victims). Thus, dogs must be very adaptable and able to settle within new environments. A third consideration for CAI teams is the intensified emotions displayed by individuals within these settings and the collective or combined emotions displayed by visitors within the setting.

All of the previous considerations require that the therapy dogs be well screened, trained, and assessed but also that handlers be especially skilled in both monitoring their dog's well-being and in working in settings and with clients with heightened emotions. Both the number of sessions and the duration of sessions in which teams work must be monitored to avoid overtaxing teams. CAI organizations must train and provide skills to handlers to equip them to process the events of the tragedy and protect their own well-being, especially as they are exposed to visitors recounting their experiences of the tragedy. Again, the collective impact of hearing, firsthand, multiple accounts of both the tragedy itself and the impact it had on individuals presents unique emotional and psychological challenges for handlers. Policies and procedures must be established by the CAI organization to monitor handler well-being after exposure to grand-scale mourning (e.g., providing access to counselors). As we've argued throughout this book, the CAI team must be screened, trained, and assessed for the work they are asked to undertake, and in the case of CAI teams supporting mourners and victims at public tragedies, the monitoring of teams during their work and upon their arrival home must be thoughtfully and carefully considered.

Homeless Shelters

To reduce agitation in residents, homeless shelters may experiment with CAIs—either by having a volunteer CAI team brought in for regularly scheduled sessions or by having a staff member bring in her or his certified therapy dog. Given the complex client profile found in this setting, the training of the CAI team is of utmost importance. The handler must be familiar with, and trained to work with, residents, many of whom may have complex mental health or addiction-related challenges. Such challenges may render the behavior of clients erratic or unpredictable. Handlers working within this context should be trained by center staff prior to attending sessions, visit the site without their dog to become familiar with the context and residents prior to beginning, and once on site liaise with and be supervised by personnel from the center.

Both handler and canine welfare must be considered within this context. The handler must closely monitor her or his dog to safeguard the dog's well-being. Client education around how best to interact with the therapy dog is important within this context, and the handler must be skilled in encouraging interactions that are not too rule bound (i.e., discouraging of interaction) yet safeguard the dog's welfare. This would include reminding clients not to feed the dog and that dogs are not to be taken out for a walk. Center personnel can help handlers in establishing boundaries around their own interactions with residents (e.g., no hugging, no gifting of objects or money). Handlers must be mindful as well of the importance of grooming before and after visits to the shelter. In light of the potentially high rates of both lice and bedbugs in homeless shelters, handlers themselves must take precautions against infestation. There appears to be low risk of human-to-dog louse infestation for the dogs themselves (AKC, 2019).

Though no published research could be found on the effects of therapy dogs within the context of a homeless shelter, gleaning findings from other contexts lends support for the notion that homeless residents would profit from spending time with therapy dogs.

Conclusion

We began this chapter by establishing the need for nuanced screening, assessment, and training of CAI teams working in specialized contexts, contexts where the demand on the CAI team may be high due to a high-stimulus environment, a complex client profile, or a high level of unpredictability. Within each of the curated examples of specialized contexts profiled in this chapter, we strove to illustrate just what it takes to ensure that CAI teams are optimally prepared for the work they're asked to undertake. As the field of CAIs expands to serve a broad and varied client base, so, too, must the screening, assessment, and training practices around identifying and preparing dog/handler teams evolve.

References

American Kennel Club (2019). *Dog lice: What they are, how to avoid them.* Retrieved January 31, 2019, from www.akc.org/expert-advice/health/can-dogs-get-lice/

Barker, S. B., Barker, R. T., McCain, N. L., & Schubert, C. M. (2016). A randomized crossover exploratory study of the effect of visiting therapy dogs on college student stress before final exams. *Anthrozoös, 29*(1), 35–46. doi: 10.1080/08927936.2015.1069988.

Binfet, J. T., Draper, Z. A., & Green, F. L. L. (in press). Stress reduction in law enforcement officers and staff through a canine-assisted intervention. *Human Animal Interaction Bulletin.*

Coren, S. (2016, February 10). Is it possible that a dog could be racist? *Psychology Today.* Retrieved from www.psychologytoday.com/us/blog/canine-corner/201602/is-it-possible-dog-could-be-racist

Crossman, M. K., Kazdin, A. E., & Knudson, K. (2015). Brief unstructured interaction with a dog reduces distress. *Anthrozoos, 28*(4), 649–659. doi: 10.1080/08927936.2015.

Fodor's Travel (2019). *12 North American airports where you can pet a therapy dog.* Retrieved from www.fodors.com/news/photos/12-north-american-airports-where-you-can-pet-a-therapy-dog

Fung, S. C. (2017). Canine-assisted reading programs for children with special educational needs: Rationale and recommendations for the use of dogs in assisting learning. Educational Review, 69, 435–450. doi: 10.1080/00131911.2016.1228611.

Hall, S. S., Gee, N. R., & Mills, D. S. (2016). Children reading to dogs: A systematic review of the literature. PLoS ONE, 11, e0149759. doi: 10.1371/journal.pone.0149759.

Hartwig, E. K., & Binfet, J. T. (2019). What's important in canine-assisted intervention teams? An investigation of canine-assisted intervention program online screening tools. *Journal of Veterinary Behavior: Clinical Applications and Research, 29,* 53–60.

Lane, H. B., & Zavada, S. D. W. (2013). When reading gets ruff: Canine-assisted reading programs. *The Reading Teacher, 67,* 87–95. doi: 10.1002/TRTR.1204.

Le Roux, M. C., Stewart, L., & Swart, E. (2014). The effect of an animal-assisted reading program on the reading rate, accuracy, and comprehension of grade 3 students: A randomized controlled study. *Child and Youth Care Forum, 43,* 655–673. doi: 10.1007/s10566-014-9262-1.

Linder, D. E., Siebens, H. C., Mueller, M., Gibbs, D. M., & Freeman, L. M. (2017). Animal-assisted interventions: A national survey of health and safety policies in hospitals, eldercare facilities, and therapy animal organizations. *American Journal of Infection Control, 45,* 883–887. doi: 10.1016/j.ajic.2017.04.287.

Pendry, P., & Vandagriff, J. L. (2019). Animal Visitation Program (AVP) reduces cortisol levels in university students: A randomized controlled trial. *AEAR Open, 5,* 1–12. doi: 10.1177/2332858419852592

Seattle Times (2017). *Nebraska dogs provide comfort after tragedies.* Retrieved from www.seattletimes.com/nation-world/nebraska-dogs-provide-comfort-after-tragedies-2/

Serpell, J. A., Coppinger, R., Fine, A. H., & Peralta, J. M. (2010). Welfare considerations in therapy and assistance animals. In A. Fine (Ed.), *Handbook on animal-assisted therapy: Theoretical foundations and guidelines for practice* (pp. 481–503). New York: Elsevier.

USA TODAY (2018). *During a tragedy a dog may be the only one to bring comfort.* Retrieved from www.usatoday.com/story/opinion/voices/2018/12/01/therapy-dogs-bring-ray-hope-during-tragedies-column/2128099002/.

Violanti, J. M., Ma, C. C., Mnatsakanova, A., Fekedulegn, D., Hartley, T. A., Gu, J. K., & Andrew, M. E. (2018). Associations between police work stressors and post-traumatic stress disorder symptoms: Examining the moderating effects of coping. *Journal of Police and Criminal Psychology.* Advance online publication. doi: 10l.1007/s11896-018-9276-y.

Ward-Griffin, E., Klaiber, P., Collins, H. K., Owens, R. L., Coren, S., & Chen, F. S. (2018). Petting away pre-exam stress: The effect of therapy dog sessions on student well-being. *Stress and Health, 34*(3), 468–473. doi: 10.1002/smi.2804.

9 Credentialing, Recredentialing, and Retirement

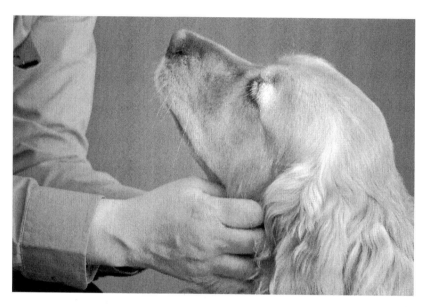

Figure 9.1 A civic employee from the Kelowna Royal Canadian Mounted Police Detachment interacts with therapy dog Dash.

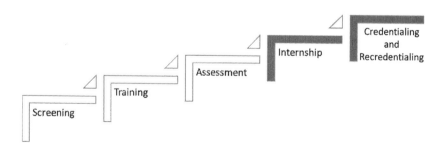

Figure 9.2 CAI team credentialing process.

Chapter 9 establishes the need for, and outlines practices to, guide the monitoring of CAI teams after their training and assessment has taken place. In this chapter we review the need for an internship for new CAI teams and describe how teams might be mentored within this stage of the credentialing process. Next, we discuss the credentialing process itself and provide an overview of the rights afforded CAI teams working on behalf of a CAI organization. We end the chapter with an overview of the recredentialing process and the need to have teams' skills and dispositions reassessed over time. As part of ensuring canine welfare, we include in this chapter an overview of when to retire a therapy dog.

Scenario

> Cheryl was thrilled when she and her dog, Charlie, were accepted into the top CAI organization in her city. Based on conversations from her dog obedience classes and from talk at her local dog park, she knew not everyone was accepted and that the agency did very thorough assessments of both handlers and their dogs. Their first placement was in a retirement facility where they supported seniors with dementia. She found this rewarding, but as Cheryl was a retired teacher, she asked they be considered for work in a teen drop-in center where teens struggling with a variety of issues could find support. The CAI organization for which Cheryl volunteered received a donation from a local drop-in center to provide a therapy dog in the waiting room as a way to increase the likelihood that teens would wait for their health care or mental health appointment. Cheryl loved her visits and could see firsthand that she and Charlie were doing important work. As their visits continued, Cheryl noticed Charlie's behavior changing and her moment of clarity came when Charlie jumped up to greet a regular visitor to the center and licked his face—behaviors he would never have done previously and behaviors that ran counter to her agency's policies around dog-client interactions. She was disappointed she'd let Charlie's once strong skills slip and she wondered if they would pass her agency's recredentialing process scheduled for next month.

Questions for Reflection and Discussion

1. How might a handlers recognize a change in their dog's skills?
2. What should handlers do to prepare for recredentialing? Is participation in sessions enough?

In our previous chapters we examined the steps and processes involved in training and assessing CAI teams working on behalf of a CAI organization to support the well-being of clients in one or more contexts. Now, we turn our attention to the need to support CAI teams after the team assessment. We will address each of the following stages of the credentialing process: (1) internship, (2) credentialing, (3) professional growth, (4) the recredentialing process, and (5) retirement.

Internship

Recall that a CAI team advancing to an internship with a CAI organization has been successfully screened to determine their initial suitability for CAI work, has attended a training session or sessions to become familiar with and practice the skills required of CAI teams working on behalf of the organization, and have successfully passed the assessments required by the CAI organization. In short, by this point in the credentialing process, unsuitable prospective teams have been identified and notified that the skills or dispositions they possess are not in alignment with those needed to work on behalf of the CAI organization. Thus, as we look toward the internship, it may be considered an evaluative stage for prospective CAI teams to become familiar with, and showcase their emerging skills in, a real-world setting under the supervision of CAI organization personnel.

As can be typical of the credentialing process experienced by CAI teams, the assessment of skills and dispositions can take place in a setting far removed from the realities of where CAI teams will actually be working. The skills displayed by CAI teams during an assessment held at a local community center might be, and are likely to be, different from the skills required in a busy afterschool program for example. The internship is composed of supervised sessions in which the CAI team works under the tutelage of either CAI organization personnel (e.g., the director, volunteer coordinator, or canine-assisted counseling [CAC] supervisor) or under the guidance of an experienced CAI team who hold a leadership position within the organization. Without an internship, handlers can be left to their own devices and find themselves doing their best to follow organization protocol when working in applied settings. Both the environment and the clients within the applied setting can present unique and unanticipated challenges for handlers and dogs, and the internship affords new teams an opportunity to ask for clarifications or to receive feedback on their skills. In short, the internship allows teams to hone their skills within a supportive framework.

Experienced Handlers: A Resource for CAI Organizations

As many CAI programs are volunteer run, resources can be scarce, and it can be the case for CAI teams, once assessed, to begin participating in programs with no direct supervision from any organization representative. An underutilized resource in many CAI organizations is the wealth of knowledge and experience found in seasoned or veteran CAI teams. Working in conjunction with organization personnel, experienced handlers have much to offer to the internship process. At the B.A.R.K. program at the University of British Columbia, we routinely tap into this wealth of knowledge by having experienced handlers participate in key roles in all aspects of the training, credentialing, and recredentialing processes. For example, experienced handlers speak at our new handler orientation, sharing their experiences and the gratification they receive from being a handler. Experienced handlers also participate, oftentimes with their dogs, in the assessment of new CAI teams (e.g., in helping ensure interdog compatibility). Similarly, in the Texas State University AAC Academy, CAC practitioners serve as guest speakers to answer questions from new practitioners-in-training, demonstrate clinical skills in practice sessions, and provide live supervision during the CAC practicum. CAI organizations are encouraged to showcase the knowledge that veteran handlers have and use this resource to inform, guide, and shape the supervision and support of new CAI teams during the internship and recredentialing assessment.

The Role of the Internship in the Credentialing Process

Once assessed, it is recommended that CAI teams only be credentialed pending the passing of a successful internship. This internship could be composed of a certain number of sessions (e.g., 10) or of a predetermined time period (e.g., 6 months) during which organization personnel monitor performance and provide feedback to handlers to strengthen their skills and ensure their performance is in accord with the organization's mission or vision and in the best interest of clients. What is key in determining the length of the internship is that sufficient opportunity to observe the CAI team in action is afforded to one or more observers from the CAI organization.

At the start of the internship, the newly assessed CAI team should begin with short visits (e.g., 20 minutes) to allow the dog to become familiar with the setting and to allow the team to build capacity. What is ideal is that during the internship, the CAI team encounters or faces a variety of stimuli characteristic of a typical placement in this setting. If, for example, there are loud vocalizations by clients who are excited to see the CAI team, then the team's reaction to this should be observed. Similarly, if the setting sees clients with restricted mobility and wheelchairs are commonplace, then it is hoped the internship affords ample opportunities to observe the dog's reaction to clients using mobility aids.

For CAC teams, the process involves more intensive work. After passing the CAC team evaluation, practitioners and their dogs participate in the CAC practicum in which they work with clients in a clinical setting with live supervision. After the CAC practicum, the internship begins as CAC practitioners introduce their therapy dog in their own private practices, school counseling settings, and mental health agencies. The CAC internship through the AAC Academy involves practitioners and their dogs facilitating one hundred 45- to 50-minute counseling sessions over the course of a minimum of 5 months. Practitioners must participate in biweekly supervision with a CAC supervisor. This training process is similar to how graduate mental health program students are trained. Once students earn their master's degree, they must facilitate a number of counseling sessions after graduation (i.e., up to 1,500 sessions in some states) under the supervision of a clinical supervisor.

The CAC internship allows CAC teams to receive supervision and support in their own respective work settings.

During CAC internship supervision, which can be offered in person or online, practitioners and the supervisor discuss case presentations, ethical dilemmas, and canine behavior and present recorded vignettes with client and/or caregiver permission. CAC practitioners who ask their dogs to participate in too many sessions, do not address canine stress during sessions, or make choices that could be potentially harmful to a client or therapy dog may not qualify to receive their credential or may need additional training and supervision. With CAC practitioners supporting clients with mental health challenges, it is crucial for practitioners to have ongoing supervision and support during this internship period and prior to receiving a credential.

In CAI settings, it is important for organization personnel who observe new CAI teams during the internship to recognize that the team is *developing* skills—that is, there may need for corrections, recommendations, or adjustments to be made to how the CAI team interacts with clients and that it is the response or the tightening of the skills by the team that is important during this time. How does the team respond to constructive feedback and is there growth in response to feedback?

Organization personnel and handlers themselves should remain hopeful and optimistic about successfully navigating the internship, especially if sound assessment practices were in place from the start in identifying strong CAI teams. Grounds for not credentialing a CAI team during the internship might include any or all of the following:

- The dog displays aggression.
- The dog is fearful in the setting during a site visit (i.e., unable to adjust to a new setting and demonstrates an elevated startle reflex).
- The dog is fearful of clients and seeks refuge behind the handler or seeks comfort or reassurance from the handler.
- A handler behaves inappropriately (e.g., uses inappropriate language, acts as a pseudo-therapist with clients without being a CAC practitioner).
- The team is disinterested in interacting with clients, and the handler shows interest only in her or his dog.
- The handler acknowledges that the work required wasn't what they thought it would be and that serving as a CAI team in this capacity is not what they're seeking.

Credentialing the CAI Team

After the completion of a successful internship, then, and only then, would a prospective CAI team receive their credential. Whether the CAI team is credentialed by a large, national-level organization or a local, community-based

Table 9.1 Guidelines for Canine-Assisted Intervention Team Behavior

Rights and Privileges	Restrictions and Limitations
1. Acknowledgment that the CAI team has met screening, training, assessment, and internship requirements for CAI work within the purview of the issuing CAI organization	1. Acknowledgement that the CAI team is not to seek or perform duties outside of their CAI team designation, including seeking privileges afforded service dogs (i.e., public access)
2. Acknowledgment that the CAI team may participate in programs and sessions in settings sanctioned and scheduled by the CAI organization who have awarded the CAI team credential	2. Recognition that despite the use of the word "therapy" in the designation, the volunteer handler is not dispensing any therapeutic advice to clients within the context of a CAI session
3. Recognition that the CAI team participates in programs or sessions with an understanding of the liability insurance covering their participation during site visits	3. Understanding that the CAI team shall not participate in programs or sessions not sanctioned by the organization

organization, it is important that the CAI organization make clear to handlers the rights and limits of the credential they have been accorded. Just as there is ample variability in the type and scale of CAI organizations, so too is there variability in both how the title "therapy dog" is bestowed upon a team by an organization and what working as a CAI team means. As a general, guiding framework, we offer the following table to guide CAI team behavior once teams have been credentialed (see Table 9.1).

Handler Code of Conduct

A lot is asked of handlers, and they certainly can have a lot to juggle once they are assigned placements in community CAI programs. One particular challenge is the negotiation of all of the stakeholders involved in, or connected to, working as a CAI handler. There are organization and program personnel to consider, the handler him- or herself, the therapy dog, the clients supported by the CAI team, and personnel who liaise at the site. In short, all of these varied stakeholders add a layer of complexity that can render participating in a community CAI program challenging. It is important to remind handlers, regardless of the organization they find themselves serving on behalf of, that there are basic tenets to uphold that will help ensure they enjoy their CAI experience, that organization personnel can count on them as a reliable handler, and that clients coming to sessions feel well supported. The following general guidelines can serve to inform the conduct of handlers serving on behalf of a CAI organization (see Table 9.2).

Table 9.2 Handler Code of Conduct

---

1. Serve as an ambassador for the CAI organization by upholding its mission or vision.
2. Monitor canine health and welfare before, during, and after site visits.
3. Honor the CAI team commitment to attend scheduled sessions and provide ample notification when the cancelation of a scheduled session is necessary.
4. Establish parameters for client behavior and safeguard client well-being within a session.
5. Participate in professional development opportunities when offered to enhance their, and their dog's, skills.
6. Maintain open communication with the organization and report safety incidents arising during site visits.

Documentation and Credentialing of CAI Teams

CAI organizations must determine how they will both document and verify the requirements for their credentialing process, as well as determine how the CAI team credential itself will be acknowledged or awarded. Key considerations in the documentation of requirements include creating a file for each team that would contain: (1) their initial CAI team screening form (see **Appendix A**); (2) their canine health screening form (see **Appendix B**); (3) confirmation of their attendance at the training session(s); (4) their CAI team assessment outcome (see **Appendix D**); and (5) verification of the successful completion of an internship.

Organizations must also identify how the CAI team credential will be awarded to teams. This might involve a ceremony that sees teams come together where handlers are given a certificate acknowledging their achievement and their dogs given either a "therapy dog vest" or scarf for identification in public. The use of vests to identify therapy dogs offer a number of distinct advantages, notably that a laminated identification tag can be attached that includes a photo of the dog/handler team, the CAI organization name can be embroidered on vests, and any sponsorship logos can be attached by having patches sewn onto the vest. If there are working and service dogs sharing the space where CAI teams will be working, the color of the vests must be carefully considered so as to avoid confusion by the public around distinguishing working dogs from therapy dogs. CAI organizations must indicate the expiry date of their credential on the credentialing certificate awarded to handlers as this will help keep track of teams needing to be recredentialed.

Recredentialing

Once a CAI team has been credentialed by an organization, there are several pathways through which teams can receive support from the CAI organization, continue to hone their skills, and maintain their credential. We recommend that CAI teams be recredentialed every 2 years. This gives teams the opportunity to participate in CAI programs for 2 years prior to applying for recredentialing. During these 2 years, we recommend that CAI organizations have processes in place to monitor and support ongoing growth of CAI teams. The pathways to recredentialing include ongoing monitoring, professional growth, and supporting documentation.

Ongoing Monitoring of CAI Teams

The first pathway and the one recommended here is that teams are routinely monitored as part of their participation in programs. Similar to the supervision provided to teams during their internship, the monitoring of teams can occur routinely over time with the scheduling of this contingent on the resources of the organization. The ongoing monitoring of teams happens in the field and in the moment when teams are participating in programs and supporting clients. This monitoring may be done by organization personnel or by a veteran CAI handler and should provide handlers with both positive and constructive feedback. Because ongoing monitoring provides handlers with regular feedback, it alleviates handlers practicing undesirable skills or interactions with clients and avoids waiting to correct CAI team behavior only when an incident or infraction is reported to the organization.

As we have discussed throughout this book, the settings in which CAI teams might find themselves working vary and can range from private practice settings to public schools and retirement homes. Such settings can be busy, rife with visual, auditory, and olfactory stimuli to which dogs must acclimate. Additionally, these settings can be densely populated and require therapy dogs to have context-specific skills in order to support clients. This all requires nuanced handling of the dog by handlers. CAI handlers, from the moment they leave the parking lot, must be keenly aware of the influence the setting potentially has on the ability of their dog to focus on the task at hand. As always, a proactive approach in which the handler anticipates the challenges to be faced (e.g., dropped food in a hallway or an overly enthusiastic client running to catch the same elevator a CAI team has just entered) is much better than a repeatedly reactive or corrective style that can erode the dog/handler relationship.

Within each of these settings, the clients who are supported by CAI teams can themselves present challenges. As just alluded to previously, overly enthusiastic clients with high energy can excite dogs (and handlers too), encouraging dogs to misbehave (e.g., jumping up to greet a client who says "Up, up!"). Once settled in a session, handlers might find clients overcome by emotion, either recalling past connections with dogs they themselves have had or in which clients let their guard down as dogs provide comfort and render them at ease. Disclosures by clients can occur, and handlers must be equipped to support clients in this way—as with CAC practitioners, or for volunteer CAI handlers—to direct clients to resources where more appropriate and tailored therapeutic support may be offered. The identification of additional resources for clients who interact with a CAI team must be identified *before* sessions are initiated, and handlers must be able to redirect clients to accessible resources in the moment, when the need can be urgent. Take, for example, a busy college campus setting in which a CAI organization is contracted to provide support to students during examinations. Should a student disclose to a handler a desire to self-harm, the handler must be familiar with mental health support on campus in order to redirect the student and ensure the student isn't at imminent risk. In CAC work, practitioners require extra training and supervision so that they are equipped to work with clients who need extra support. Yet even CAC practitioners may need to seek out consultation from supervisors to discuss challenging client situations and ensure they can effectively support clients' emotional needs with a therapy dog.

The aforementioned complexities reveal the range of situations and clients that handlers must negotiate. As Ng and colleagues (2015, p. 370) argue, "The handlers should be continuously monitored to address problems as they occur." Without organization personnel monitoring the degree to which handlers navigate these challenges, handlers are left to self-evaluate—to monitor the extent to which they are able to adequately uphold policy and practice within the context of busy applied settings.

An additional complexity arises when organizations do not monitor on an ongoing basis the CAI teams serving on their behalf. Handlers are left to assess their dog's well-being during sessions. Are handlers able to identify indicators of stress in their dog that warrant the termination of a visit? How do handlers remember all of the policies, and potentially changing policies, of CAI organizations? As we discussed in Chapter 4, handlers may be reluctant to admit that the placement is not working or that their dog is poorly suited to the program for fear of appearing incompetent.

Monitoring Sessions

An outside set of eyes on CAI teams can be invaluable in keeping behavioral guidelines upheld and in tightening skills in need of remediation. Routine visits by organization personnel allow for the careful and ongoing monitoring of handler skills vis-à-vis their management of their dog and vis-à-vis their interactions with the public. Organization personnel are able to identify areas for handlers to address that will strengthen their handling and interaction skills. Handlers, for example, can be reminded of how to position their dog in ways that encourage optimal opportunities for clients to interact or might be reminded to set limits for clients (e.g., no picking up dogs), especially in situations where the CAI team visits the same clients repeatedly and clients, through familiarity with the dog, may overstep boundaries. The routine monitoring of handlers in real-world applied settings also allows organization personnel to assess the extent to which CAI teams uphold policy and serve as ambassadors for the organization. A poorly groomed dog arriving to a hospital with a heavy choke collar who eats dropped food while en route to a session can do harm to an organization's reputation within the community.

Reevaluation of CAI Teams

Another option for ongoing monitoring is reevaluation of CAI teams. Some organizations require teams to be reassessed by participating and passing another CAI team assessment, as outlined in Chapter 7, in order to remain credentialed with the organization. CAI organizations can schedule these team assessments at recredentialing time, every 2 years. Organizations who choose to reevaluate teams would facilitate the CAI team assessment in the same way as the initial team assessment. If teams pass the assessment, then teams would then be eligible to continue the recredentialing process. If teams do not pass the evaluation, then CAI organizations can consider how to best support the handler and therapy dog in deciding the required next steps. This may involve providing additional training and/or additional mentorship by a veteran CAI team within the organization before allowing the team to be reevaluated.

Professional Growth for CAI Teams

In our experience running large CAI and CAC programs we have found handlers eager to participate in postcredentialing educational opportunities. In fact, such sessions are often welcomed by handlers. It gives handlers a chance to meet one another and network, provide feedback on the delivery of programs, raise challenges faced out in the field during site visits, and share strategies or techniques they've found effective in their handling of their dog or in interactions with clients. We recommend that CAI organizations offer continuing education for all teams and require teams to complete a minimum of 3 hours of ongoing training every year, as part of recredentialing requirements (i.e., attending one half-day workshop). This means that handlers would be required to obtain 6 hours of continuing education every 2 years in order to be eligible for recredentialing.

Topics for handler training sessions might include the following (see Table 9.3).

Table 9.3 Professional Development Topics for Handlers

Topic	Description of Seminar
Recent developments in the field	As many handlers may not have formal training in the field of HAI, this session can provide handlers with an overview of the benefits of HAIs and recent findings attesting to the benefits of CAI work. Programs operating in urban centers might consider inviting a researcher from their local university who works in the area of HAI to be a guest speaker.

(Continued)

Table 9.3

Topic	Description of Seminar
Connecting with clients	This can be an interactive workshop in which experienced handlers in the program are invited to help craft and deliver a session to showcase strategies handlers can use to connect with clients during sessions. This might include a review of what information to share with clients about themselves and their dogs, questions to ask clients, and information to share about the program in general. Workshops can be thematically organized and may, for example, address working with children and teens.
Conditions for an optimal canine visit	This session can provide an overview for handlers around the conditions that contribute to a dog/handler team having a positive or optimal session. This might include the role of exercising a dog prior to a visit, the role (or restriction) of treats during visits, how to keep dogs focused on human clients when other therapy dogs are present, and how to position dogs within sessions to encourage client interactions.
How to actively listen to clients	Clarifying the role of handlers is key to ensuring the successful participation of dog/handler teams within programs. This session can review the role of the handler and strategies that handlers can use to actively engage with, and listen to, clients (e.g., the use of open versus closed prompts).
Setting boundaries for clients and client education	Informing or educating clients about what to expect and how to behave during a session is an often-overlooked aspect of CAI. This session can provide handlers with strategies around interacting with therapy dogs, including the dos and don'ts for a session.
Monitoring canine well-being: understanding indicators of canine stress	Ideally handlers would have received information on the indicators of canine stress during their initial orientation and training session with the agency. As a refresher and in the event this was not shared, a session may be held that provides handlers with an overview of the key signs of canine stress. Conversely, signs of positive adjustment by dogs in sessions should also be reviewed (e.g., how you know your dog is settling in a session).
Advanced handler skills	This session can provide handlers with an overview of the skills that they can develop and that their dogs can develop to enhance their participation in CAIs. For handlers, advanced skills might include how to redirect a client in distress to additional, outside resources or how to create a microcommunity of support when multiple clients are simultaneously interacting with a dog. For therapy dogs, this might include learning to place their head on the shoulder of a client to simulate a hug, to approach the side of a wheelchair and await a cue to place a paw on the armrest, or to accept prolonged eye contact.
Handler opportunities within the program	Handlers appreciate being kept informed of developments within the organization for which they volunteer. This session might include providing handlers with an overview of new handler opportunities within the organization or information regarding new initiatives (e.g., fundraising needs).

Table 9.3 (Continued)

Topic	Description of Seminar
Supervising new CAI teams	This session is for veteran CAI handlers who are interested in supporting new CAI teams through ongoing monitoring and supervision. This professional development opportunity can teach handlers how to conduct supervised visits of new CAI teams, what challenges or concerns to look for, how to recognize team strengths, and how to provide feedback to teams who struggle. For CAC teams, supervisors need to be trained as clinical supervisors in mental health prior to becoming CAC team supervisors. CAC supervision training can focus on identifying strengths and areas for growth for CAC team clinical skills and supporting CAC teams through ethical dilemmas, complex client issues, and how to advocate for the client and therapy dog concurrently.
Becoming a CAI team evaluator	Having qualified CAI team evaluators working on their behalf is essential for CAI organizations. Organizations should offer a training in which potential CAI team evaluators can practice facilitating individual team evaluation skills (e.g., asking a team to do the *come when called* skill and then scoring that skill under the tutelage of an experienced team evaluator). Then potential team evaluators can practice facilitating a full CAI team assessment with volunteer teams.
Supporting the grieving client	This session can provide handlers with skills and resources for supporting grieving clients in various settings, such as hospice work and crisis response. This session can teach handlers information about the grieving process and veteran CAI teams with experience in grief work could demonstrate skills needed to support grieving clients.

The Recredentialing Process

In our own review of CAI organizations and in scanning reports of other researchers working in this area, it certainly appears that the requirement of recredentialing for CAI teams is not standard practice in the field (Hartwig & Binfet, 2019). Recall the work of Linder, Siebens, Mueller, Gibbs, and Freeman (2017) who, in their survey of CAI organizations, found one third of programs required only the American Kennel Club Canine Good Citizen certificate in order for a CAI team to be credentialed for participation in canine therapy. Also troubling is that in many cases, once CAI teams are credentialed, this determination that the CAI team is of sound character and possesses the necessary skills and dispositions to serve in community programs to support the well-being of clients holds for the duration of the handler's tenure with an organization.

We argue here that this is insufficient, especially in light of all of the variation in screening, training, and assessment practices evident across CAI organizations. It merits noting that if suboptimal initial assessment practices are implemented by an organization (e.g., merely requiring a Canine Good

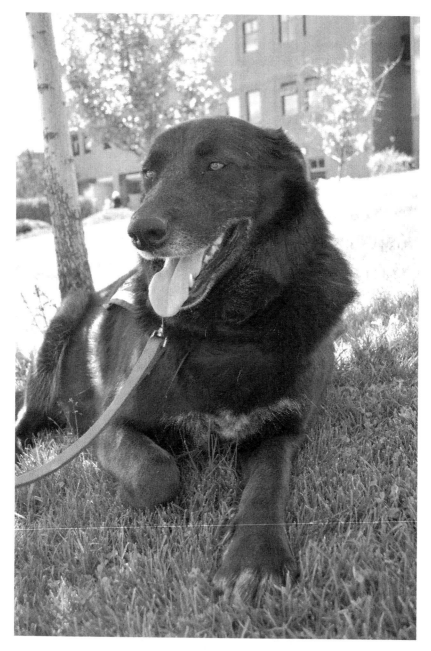

Figure 9.3 Therapy dog Siska taking a break from a session.

Citizen certificate), then repeatedly demanding this same assessment over time will not be informative of CAI team competency and would serve little purpose. However, where comprehensive CAI team assessment practices are in place at the outset and the ongoing, routine monitoring of teams during site visits is not done, the recredentialing of handlers should be done every 2 years after the initial credential is received.

The recredentialing process for CAI teams seeking to continue volunteering on behalf of a CAI organization should involve: (1) the submission of a short application indicating the team is requesting to be recertified, (2) the submission of an updated canine health screening form akin to the one submitted during the team's initial application for certification with the organization, (3) the submission of an updated criminal record check, and (4) the payment of any fees pending the organization's policies for the assessment and reassessment of teams. As part of the application process for recredentialing, there must be an opportunity for handlers to disclose information regarding any changes in their dog's health or any behavioral incidents that have taken place since the initial credentialing occurred.

The need to recredential CAI teams has certainly been acknowledged in the field (e.g., Ng et al., 2015) and is founded on the recognition that dog temperament and disposition can change over time, thus necessitating an ongoing credentialing process. If CAI teams who have been credentialed for a particular setting (e.g., a counseling clinic) are asked to serve in a new setting with a new client population (e.g., to children who are reluctant readers in an elementary school), then reassessment and training is required. This is done to ensure that the CAI team is well suited to the new setting and new client population and helps ensure best safety practices are upheld. We now turn our attention to factors that help determine when a therapy dog should retire.

Retirement

Determining when both handlers and therapy dogs should retire from CAI work is an important decision. CAI work can be extremely rewarding, both personally and professionally, but it can also be demanding depending on the client population served. Next, we'll explore considerations around the retirement of handlers and dogs.

Handler Retirement

Handlers could potentially volunteer in a CAI organization or provide CAI services for several years. Over time, handlers may find themselves working with several therapy dogs, all of whom must be assessed and credentialed with the handler, during the handler's tenure with an organization. Like all volunteer work, the decision to retire from CAI work should be made by the handler in discussion with CAI organization personnel. If actively participating in programs becomes too taxing for a handler, there may be administrative opportunities within the organization that allow the handler to continue contributing, albeit indirectly, to supporting client well-being.

Therapy Dog Retirement

Building on the work of Urfer and colleagues (2011), Binfet, Silas, Longfellow, and Widmaier-Waurechen (2018) noted that the average life span across breeds was determined to be 12.2 years (*SD* = 1.97; range 7–16.5 years). As a general rule, smaller dogs tend to live longer than larger breed dogs, and there is ample variability in the life span of different canine breeds (Adams, Evans, Sampson, & Wood, 2010; Adams, Morgan, & Watson, 2018; Bonnett, Egenvall, Hedhammar, & Olson, 2005; Galis, Van Der Sluijs, van Dooren, Metz, & Nussbaumer, 2007; O'Neill, Church, McGreevy, Thomson, & Brodbelt, 2013; Wallis, Szabo, Erdelyi-Belle, & Kubinyi, 2018). The question of when a therapy dog should retire can be informed by canine life span science. Recognizing that working as a therapy dog can be taxing (envision for a moment the skills required by a therapy dog working in a busy airport to reduce travelers' stress), one must ask if the dog is robust enough and able to withstand the environmental stressors found within her or his working environment. Should the retirement age of therapy dogs be determined on a case-by-case basis or should CAI organizations establish a predetermined retirement age as a blanket policy?

Research on Canine Aging: When Is a Dog Old?

In scouring the literature on canine aging, health, and behavior, a few key findings emerge that inform our understanding around indicators suggesting it is time for a therapy dog to retire. Particularly relevant to our discussion is how the temperament of a dog potentially changes with age. Across studies, researchers have identified that human-dog interactions can be age sensitive (e.g., Baranyiova, Holub, Tyrlik, Janackova, & Ernstova, 2004; Salman et al., 2000; Salvin, McGreevy, Sachdev, & Valenzuela, 2011). In their study of the life span of pet dogs, researchers Lisa Wallis and colleagues (2018, p. 2) write,

> Aging in dogs is also associated with a decline in perceptual and cognitive functions. These declines may result in problematic behavioral changes, ranging from increased vocalization, aggression and phobias, to a loss in house training, which may affect the quality of life of the individual and the human-animal bond.

Thus, though therapy dogs certainly gain experience over time, becoming "seasoned veterans" of hospital or college campus programs, their ability to withstand the stressors inherent in these environments can be compromised with advancing age. Handlers (and organization personnel) are responsible for the constant monitoring of canine welfare, of which the assessment of older dogs' enjoyment of and capacities to work must be routinely evaluated. No published research on the longevity of therapy dogs was identified, but if dogs are certified on average at 2–3 years and retired somewhere around age 10, canine agencies can expect CAI teams to provide support to clients for 7 or 8 years.

In a study exploring how participation in CAI impacts therapy dogs, McCullough and colleagues (2018) provide a description of the therapy dogs who participated in their study. In addition to describing the breeds and gender of the dogs, they indicate that dogs aged 2 to 13 participated in the study. Here we find an example of a 13-year-old therapy dog who is working in a robust capacity and actively contributing to research. Very likely, this dog had ample prior experience, was accustomed to working in the setting and with the target population, and was closely monitored by her or his handler throughout study protocols.

Given the variability in the life span of dogs and the variability in temperamental changes as dogs age, a decision to retire a therapy dog should be made in consultation with the dog's veterinarian, the dog's handler, and representatives from the CAI organization. Certainly, a review of the dog's recent performance over time would be a strong indicator of the dog's ability to continue working (e.g., has the dog shown a change in her or his ability to withstand stressors in the working environment?). Discussion of the following guidelines can collectively assist caregivers and stakeholders in determining the retirement age of individual therapy dogs and the working conditions of older therapy dogs.

Guidelines for Monitoring Older Therapy Dogs

1. The dog is determined to be in optimal health by her or his veterinarian. It is important that CAI organizations require handlers submit a recent canine health screening form when applying for recredentialing.
2. Though the dog might slow down, he or she continues to appear enjoying providing support to the public. Should this be the case, might shorter visits be booked for this CAI team?
3. The handler is aware of, and monitors, the frequency and intensity of age-related changes in temperament, including changes in baseline behavior around vocalizations, aggression, phobias, and startle reflex.
4. The therapy dog's age is a consideration in the CAI team's participation in community programs (e.g., older dogs may be better suited to clients with quiet profiles and in quiet settings).
5. In seeing signs of physical aging indicating retirement is approaching, organizations restrict the number and duration of CAI team visits and restricts the number of clients per session for older therapy dogs.

This section on canine retirement emphasizes the importance of supporting canine welfare throughout their participation in a CAI program and beyond.

We encourage handlers to always consider what is best for their dog, even if it means their dog must withdraw from participating in programs that provided support to clients and brought joy to the handler.

Conclusion

The aim of this chapter was to illustrate and emphasize the importance of credentialing, recredentialing, and retirement of CAI teams by a CAI organization. One strong theme in our book has been that CAI teams must be comprehensively screened, trained, and assessed prior to being credentialed. We also emphasize that CAI organizations need stronger compliance in their use of rigorous screening, training, assessment, and monitoring methods when credentialing and recredentialing teams. Doing so helps ensure that CAI team skills, behaviors, and dispositions are in alignment with both the client and context needs.

References

Adams, V. J., Evans, K. M., Sampson, J., & Wood, J. L. N. (2010). Methods and mortality results of a health survey of purebred dogs in the UK. *Journal of Small Animal Practice, 51*, 512–524. doi: 10.1111/j.1748-5827.2010.00974.x.

Adams, V. J., Morgan, D. M., & Watson, P. (2018). Healthy ageing and the science of longevity in dogs. Part I: Is grey the new gold? *Companion Animal, 23*, 12–17. doi: 10.12968/coan.2018.23.1.12.

Baranyiova, E., Holub, A., Tyrlik, M., Janackova, B., & Ernstova, M. (2004). Behavioural differences in dogs of various ages in Czech households. *Acta Veterinaria Brno, 73*, 229–233. doi: 10.2754/avb200473020229.

Binfet, J. T., Silas, H. J., Longfellow, S. W., & Widmaier-Waurechen, K. (2018). When veterinarians support canine therapy: Bidirectional benefits for clinics and therapy programs. *Veterinary Sciences, 5*, 1–8. doi: 10-.3390/vetsci5010002.

Bonnett, B. N., Egenvall, A., Hedhammar, A., & Olson, P. (2005). Mortality in over 350,000 insured Swedish dogs from 1995–2000: Breed-, gender-, age-and cause-specific rates. *Acta Veterinaria Scandinavica, 46*, 105–120. doi: 10.1186/1751-0147-46-105.

Galis, F., Van Der Sluijs, I., van Dooren, T. J. M., Metz, J. A. J., & Nussbaumer, M. (2007). Do large dogs die young? *Journal of Experimental Zoology, 308B*, 119–126. doi: 10.1002/jez.b.21116.

Hartwig, E., & Binfet, J. T. (2019). What's important in canine-assisted intervention teams? An investigation of canine-assisted intervention program online screening tools. *Journal of Veterinary Behavior: Clinical Applications and Research, 29*, 53–60.

Linder, D. E., Siebens, H. C., Mueller, M., Gibbs, D. M., & Freeman, L. M. (2017). Animal-assisted interventions: A national survey of health and safety policies in hospitals, eldercare facilities, and therapy animal organizations. *American Journal of Infection Control, 45*, 883–887. doi: 10.1016/j.ajic.2017.04.287.

McCullough, A., Jenkins, M. A., Ruehrdanz, A., Gilmer, M. J., Olson, J. . . . O'Haire, M. (2018). Physiological and behavioral effects of animal-assisted interventions on therapy dogs in pediatric oncology settings. *Applied Animal Behaviour Science, 200*, 86–95. doi: 10.1016/j.applanim.2017.11.014.

Ng, Z., Albright, J., Fine, A. H., & Peralta, J. (2015). Our ethical and moral responsibility: Ensuring the welfare of therapy animals. In A. H. Fine (Ed.), *Handbook on animal-assisted therapy: Foundations and guidelines for animal-assisted interventions* (pp. 357–376). New York: Elsevier.

O'Neill, D. G., Church, D. B., McGreevy, P. D., Thomson, P. C., & Brodbelt, D. C. (2013). Longevity and mortality of owned dogs in England. *Veterinary Journal, 198*, 638–643. doi: 10.1016/j.tvjl.2013.09.020.

Salman, M. D., Hutchinson, J., Ruch-Gallie, R., Kogan, L., New, J. C., Kass, P. H., & Scarlett, J. M. (2000). Behavioural reasons for relinquishment of dogs and cats to 12 shelters. *Journal of Applied Animal Welfare Science, 3*, 93–106. doi: 10.1207/S15327604JAWS0302_2.

Salvin, H. E., McGreevy, P. D., Sachdev, P. S., & Valenzuela, M. J. (2011). Growing old gracefully: Behavioral changes associated with "successful aging" in the dog, Canis familiaris. *Journal of Veterinary Behavior, 6*, 313–320. doi: 10.1016/j.jveb.2011.04.004.

Urfer, S. R., Greer, K., & Wolf, N. S. (2011). Age related cataract in dogs: A biomarker for life span and its relation to body size. *Age, 33*, 451–460. doi: 10.1007/s11357-010-9158-4.

Wallis, L. J., Szabo, D., Erdelyi-Belle, B., & Kubinyi, E. (2018). Demographic change across the lifespan of pet dogs and their impact on health status. *Frontiers in Veterinary Science, 5*, 1–20. doi: 10.3389/fvets.2018.00200.

10 Future Directions in Canine-Assisted Interventions

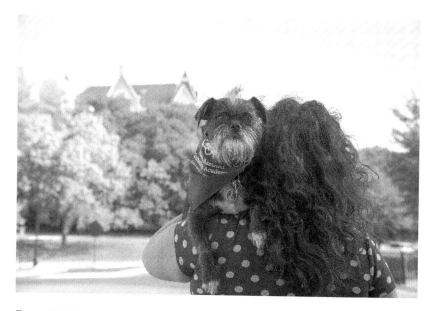

Figure 10.1 Future directions with CAC practitioner Wanda Montemayor and therapy dog Chango.

The aim of this last chapter is to explore new directions and innovations in the field of CAIs. Certainly, one theme throughout this book has been highlighting the variability that exists within the field of CAI, including variations in language and in how CAI teams are screened, trained, assessed, and credentialed. Our hope is that our book has helped clarify and reduce some of this variability, and the topics that follow in this chapter are offered to both continue this clarification process and to provoke the thinking of readers around the future delivery of CAIs. This chapter will be especially useful to practitioners and researchers wanting to keep abreast of new developments in the field. It is hoped that the information that follows inspires both applied work in varied contexts and research that contributes to our understanding of the benefits of CAIs for human well-being.

Scenario

Alice is the director of a local CAI organization called Paws for Children. Her organization has 12 teams who provide CAI services to children with special needs in schools. Alice has developed this program over the past 5 years in her extra time outside of her full-time job as a librarian. For Paws for Children, Alice has created a volunteer application and a 3-hour handler training and has partnered with Canine Good Citizen evaluators to assess and credential her teams. The Paws for Children teams have enjoyed working with children, yet several issues have arisen over the past few years. Alice had to dismiss one handler who was allowing children to hug the dog for long periods of time, after which, on one occasion, the dog growled at a child. Alice has also noticed that some of her handlers allow children to interact with the dogs while the handlers talk among each other. Alice realizes that some of her teams may need supplementary training and that Paws for Children likely needs stronger practices around the training and assessment of basic CAI team skills and specific skills needed in school settings with children. In July, while at a conference, Alice had the opportunity to participate in a workshop on CAI team credentialing. After learning more about CAI research and credentialing standards, Alice realizes that she needs to enhance her screening, training, and assessment protocols for preparing teams for CAI work.

Questions for Reflection and Discussion

1. What resources could Alice use to improve screening, training, and assessment protocols used in Paws for Children?
2. How can Alice identify and connect with other CAI organizations who are doing similar work?
3. How can researchers, educators, and other CAI organizations help inform the work of programs like Paws for Children?

Best Practices for CAI Teams

One way to move the CAI field forward is for all CAI organizations to use best practices. Our book has explored CAI team screening, training, assessment, and credentialing. In each chapter we have supported our recommendations for preparing and credentialing CAI teams with references to human-animal interaction (HAI) literature. In what follows, we summarize and provide an overview of our recommendations for best practices for credentialing CAI teams (see Table 10.1).

As CAI researchers, educators, and organizations adopt best practices and standards for the field, this unifies and strengthens the integrity of the CAI field.

Table 10.1 Best Practices for Credentialing CAI Teams Overview

Chapter	Content Area	CAI Best Practices
1	CAI terminology	Using consistent terminology in the field of HAI and CAI
2	Types of CAIs	Using consistent terminology for CAI practices: CAA, CAE, CAT, and CAC
3	CAI team screening	Using a standardized screening form for potential CAI teams that includes the following: • basic information • motivation to volunteer • handler/dog relationship • temperament • previous volunteer or work experience • previous experience with animals • training • background check • equipment used or needed • availability
3	Additional screening criteria	Employing policies and additional screening criteria for the following: • handler and canine hygiene • canine health, vaccinations, and diet • canine temperament and skills • handler temperament and skills
4	CAI team welfare	Educating handlers to do the following: • recognize, interpret, and respond to canine communication (i.e., positive behavior and stress signals) • limit the number and length of CAI sessions • consider when to terminate sessions • educate clients about CAI and canine behavior
5	CAI team knowledge training	Ensuring handlers are trained in the following: • CAI program basics • handler and therapy dog job descriptions • facility or practice logistics • safety/incident report procedures • reporting success stories
5	Training philosophy	Promoting positive reinforcement and prohibiting aversive training techniques for CAI teams
5	Canine socialization	Ensuring that puppies and potential therapy dogs have sufficient socialization with diverse people, places, and sounds

Chapter	Content Area	CAI Best Practices
5	CAI team prerequisites	Requiring the CGC test or a similar basic obedience prerequisite prior to CAI team training and assessment and also not using the CGC test as a proxy for CAI team assessment
5	CAI team skills training and practice	Teaching and providing practice opportunities for the following CAI team skills prior to the team evaluation:
		• handler check-in • accepting a friendly stranger • teaching how to greet a dog • sit • handling • down • grooming • walking on a loose leash • walking through a crowd • managing several people who want to pet the dog • reaction to distractions • reaction to a team with a neutral dog • stay and come when called • setting a limit—restraining hug • setting a limit—request to take dog • leave it • accepting a treat
6	CAC team training	Ensuring CAC teams have training and competencies in the following areas:
		• CAC history and theory application • CAC techniques • CAC treatment planning • CAC case conceptualization • CAC team evaluation—evaluating CAC teams for skills specific to clinical settings with clients • CAC practicum—using the CAC skills checklist to develop and hone clinical skills with a therapy dog • CAC supervision
7	CAI team assessment preparation	Preparing for team assessments by considering the following:
		• room setup • volunteers • how to reduce team stress level • approved and restricted equipment/resources
7	CAI team assesment skills	Assessing teams on the same skills on which they were trained and have had practice (see Chapter 5 CAI team skills)

(Continued)

Table 10.1 (Continued)

Chapter	Content Area	CAI Best Practices
8	Specialized CAI contexts	Providing training and assessment for specialized skills in the following contexts: • schools • college campuses • police precincts • hospitals • airports • crisis response settings
9	Internship	Requiring an internship for CAI teams prior to team credentialing
9	Credentialing	Having a clear credentialing and recredentialing process in place
9	Professional growth	Offering continuing education opportunities for CAI teams

Future Directions for CAI Organizations

International Database of CAI Organizations

As we look to what's needed in the field, one source of the variability in how CAI teams are screened, trained, and assessed is found in the sheer number of CAI organizations in operation. Each with its own mission or vision that guides their delivery of programs, these organizations range from large-scale organizations with correspondingly large budgets and sponsors to small, community-driven organizations with limited scope and reach. What is currently missing in the field is an international database to document the CAI organizations in existence. Establishing an international database of CAI organizations would help coalesce efforts underway by different organizations, offer support to fledgling organizations, and assist clients in their search for access to CAI teams. An international database would allow organizations to record their contact information; year established; locations and clients served; their screening, training, and assessment practices; and the number of CAI teams they credential annually. One example of a system for tracking organization information is an online database called GuideStar (2018). GuideStar gathers and distributes information about nonprofit organizations with a mission to "revolutionize philanthropy by providing information that advances transparency, enables users to make better decisions, and encourages charitable giving" (para. 6). The GuideStar database is composed of 2.7 million nonprofits with 26 million annual searches for information. Similar to GuideStar, an international database for CAI organizations would provide people, companies, and funders with opportunities to learn about, donate to, volunteer with, and partner with different CAI organizations. Establishing a worldwide gathering place for CAI organizations holds promise and is needed to advance the field.

The Establishment of a CAI Governing Body

In this book we have coalesced skills and dispositions that best prepare CAI teams for successful interactions with client. What is now needed in the field is the establishment of an international governing body to oversee CAI organizations worldwide. An international governing body would help to reduce variability through the identification of shared standards that may be upheld across contexts to identify CAI teams. This governing body would distinguish the important work of therapy dogs across varied contexts, as well as foster transparency for prospective handlers, organizations, and clients. The CAI governing body could be comprised of a 10-member board of directors. The 10 members could include a CEO, chair, past chair, chair-elect, secretary, and five other board member positions. The governing body, in turn, could develop a governance manual that provides the following definitions and policies:

- mission
- ends policies (i.e., goals and expected outcomes of the governing body)
- board member job descriptions, selection procedures, code of conduct, and officer roles
- CEO job description, compensation, and succession process
- board committee governance principles and structure
- monitoring procedures and reports

It is crucial that the governing body is composed of board members who represent the varied practices of CAI, as well as have members from different countries, CAI roles (e.g., researchers, educators, and administrators), and organizations.

The governing body could develop committees devoted to the enhancement of CAI standards in the following categories:

- education and training
- research
- ethics and practices
- leadership
- organization accreditation

These committees could be led by the CEO and select board members and could be composed of CAI handlers and practitioners who have experience and passion for developing and enriching specific areas in the CAI field. For example, members of the research committee could be composed of the CEO, a board member, three CAI researchers, and two students and have a goal of developing a research protocol for CAI research in schools. These committees would allow more local members to be involved in the governing body while still being led and guided by elected board members.

The governing body could also provide opportunities for members to be involved in the development of new policies and standards for the field. The development of a CAI leadership program, facilitated by the governing body, would allow administrators, educators, researchers, handlers, and practitioners interested in being more involved in CAI leadership to participate in a training program to prepare future leaders of the field. This training program would offer a pipeline to the committees listed previously, so that each year committees could have a combination of experienced and new members serving.

We believe that the development of a governing body is an important next step in our field and would set the stage for the ability to accredit CAI organizations.

Accreditation of CAI Organizations

"Consequently, numerous animal-assisted activity and animal-assisted therapy organizations set their own guidelines and regulations, making standardization of the field difficult" (Ng, Albright, Fine, & Peralta, 2015, p. 357). When we consider that, for the most part, CAI organizations are run by administrators with varied training and expertise in human and canine behavior and possibly limited training in HAI research and canine behavior, combined with a lack of field standards both in the screening and assessment of CAI team skills, we see there is a need for the assessment of CAI organizations. How might an organization know it is meeting minimum standards of practice for humans and for dogs without feedback from someone outside the organization who can attest to the extent to which best practices are upheld and met?

Just as establishing a governing body to oversee CAI organizations and the development of CAI screening, training, and assessment standards helps unite the field of CAIs, might there be future calls for CAI organizations to be accredited? As the popularity of CAIs grows and CAI organizations are asked to provide CAI teams for work in new contexts to support new and diverse clients, the accreditation of an organization helps the public discern the extent to which an organization has adhered to the tenets of best practice. We recommend the following categories and applied examples for the development of accreditation standards (see Table 10.2).

Table 10.2 CAI Organization Accreditation Categories and Examples

Accreditation Categories	Applied Examples
CAI organization	• Organizations are registered on the international database of CAI organizations. • Organizations have an active website. • Organizations adopt a code of ethics to promote the integrity of the CAI field. • Directors and administrators have documented training in CAI services, canine behavior, and HAI literature. • Organizations agree to abide by standards adopted by national or international accrediting entities.

Table 10.2 (Continued)

Accreditation Categories	Applied Examples
Screening	• Organizations have a screening process in place that identifies teams that would be a good fit for CAI work and teams who are not a match for CAI services.
Training	• Organizations have a basic obedience prerequisite in place prior to team training. • Organizations offer sufficient training and practice for CAI teams prior to a team evaluation.
Assessment	• Organizations use a consistent CAI team assessment procedure that assesses teams for basic and advanced team skills, reactions to diverse clients, and skills for specialized contexts.
Credentialing	• Organizations support teams during an internship prior to credentialing teams. • Organizations have a credentialing and recredentialing protocol in place. • Organizations offer continuing education for CAI teams.

CAI organization accreditation would increase the integrity of our field by ensuring that all CAI organizations meet minimum standards for CAI team preparation and credentialing.

Future Directions in CAI Research

Just as the number and iterations of CAIs has flourished, so, too, has there been a corresponding proliferation in empirical work done to investigate the experience of, and the effects of, spending time with therapy dogs. In our opening chapter we acknowledged the concerns raised by researchers (e.g., Crossman, 2017; Crossman, Kazdin, Matijczak, Kitt, & Santos, 2018; Herzog, 2011, 2014; Marino, 2012) around the need for increased scientific rigor when investigating HAIs.

As research advances, quantitative researchers would be wise to ensure that research designs include randomization for treatment and control conditions after the administration of pretest measures, that power analyses are conducted a priori to ensure sample sizes are sufficiently robust, that follow-up measures are administered after posttest measures to assess the extent to which findings have long lasting impact (i.e., "stick"), and that triangulated data collection is used to increase the reliability of findings.

In qualitative research, especially when the voice of participants is captured through interviews, it remains important for researchers to justify their sample size, follow systematic analytic procedures when making sense of participant-generated data and be mindful of saturation when coding responses, consider within-case and across-case analyses where appropriate, incorporate member checking and member reflections as part of the methodology, and report inter-rater agreement when participants' responses are thematically coded.

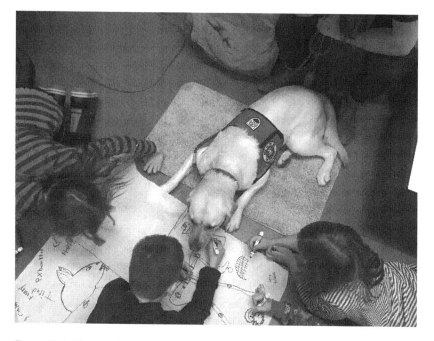

Figure 10.2 Therapy dog Amber supports children in an after-school leadership program at the University of British Columbia.

Regardless of the methodological approach undertaken, researchers are encouraged to design studies that capture multivocality (i.e., ratings, perceptions, or viewpoints of handlers, clients, and CAI organization personnel). There has been an abundance of research exploring the effects of CAIs on outcomes in clients, some research examining the impact on therapy dogs themselves, and little research exploring the impact of CAIs on handlers. As we illustrated in Chapter 1, there remains a need to conduct research across all the contexts within which we see CAI teams working.

Recommendations for Researchers

Beyond the aforementioned research considerations, our broader recommendations for researchers working with CAI teams include (1) reporting the mean age and experience of the therapy dogs participating in research and avoid using newly credentialed dog/handler teams, (2) reporting canine welfare protocols as part of the Procedures section of their publications, (3) reporting the CAI team-to-client ratio as an indication of the working conditions therapy dogs experienced, and (4) reporting the total number of sessions and the duration of sessions.

The goal of many researchers is to advance science or knowledge around a particular topic and inform practice. This theory-to-practice bridge is important in identifying evidence-based best practices. There are, however, challenges that arise in the extrapolation of study findings to applied community programming. Within the context of CAIs these challenges might include but are not limited to the following:

1. How knowledge is disseminated to practitioners. Knowledge translation strategies must be upheld so that scientific findings are not "cherry picked" to sway practice. Just how might community practitioners interested in CAI access research findings that hold potential to inform their programs?
2. Studies are done on specific populations and findings identified in one population do not necessarily transfer to, and are not applicable to, other populations (e.g., studies done on adult participants may have limited applicability to child populations).
3. Many CAI studies are done employing small sample sizes that makes generalizability problematic.
4. Studies employ a predetermined team-to-client ratio when significant findings are found. This ratio must be considered in applied contexts.
5. The working conditions for therapy dogs in experimental designs are often not the same as working conditions found in real-world, applied settings.
6. The experimental rigor used in many studies may be lacking (i.e., no randomization to control condition, poorly conceived control conditions).
7. There is a potential confounding of findings when different animals are used (i.e., equine findings inform beliefs around CAI effectiveness).
8. There is a lack of clarity around the mechanisms of CAIs that contribute to human well-being (i.e., is ambient interaction sufficient or is hands-on interaction required?).
9. Bias may be evident when researchers, interested in and predisposed to believing CAIs have a positive impact on human well-being, do not take precautions to reduce researcher bias.

Reducing researcher bias, though an oft-overlooked dimension of HAI research, is especially important for research in the field of CAIs, where researchers themselves are likely to be dog lovers and may be predisposed to believe there are benefits to spending time with therapy dogs. As Griffin and colleagues (2011, p. 6) argue, "HAI (human-animal interaction) research tends to be conducted by animal lovers, who may be biased toward finding positive HAI effects." Thus, researchers would be wise to take steps to reduce bias and report, as part of their routine procedural description within manuscripts, the steps that were taken to reduce this bias while conducting research on the benefits of therapy canines. Such steps might include not using their own animals in interventions, using random assignment to treatment and control conditions where applicable as mentioned earlier, and always using credentialed dog/handler teams in protocols.

Conclusion

This chapter explored future directions in CAIs. We provided an overview of best practices for CAI team credentialing. We also identified the need for an international database of CAI organizations. One key recommendation we made is the establishment of a CAI governing body, composed of a board of directors and committees devoted to advancing specific CAI areas. We also

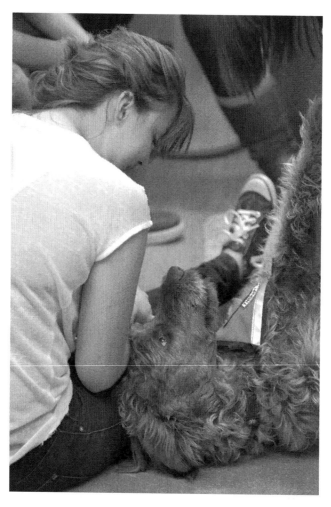

Figure 10.3 A tender moment between a college student and a therapy dog from the B.A.R.K. program.

see the development of an accreditation process of CAI organizations as a future goal for this field. Last, we made recommendations for future directions in CAI research.

As researchers and practitioners working in the field of CAIs, we have seen firsthand how therapy dogs can positively influence the lives of clients across a variety of contexts. The impact of therapy dogs can be enhanced when dogs are a part of a well-trained and credentialed CAI team. We hope our passion for this field and our recommendations of best practices and pathways will advance your own work with therapy dogs—whether you're a handler keen to share your dog with the public; the director of a CAI organization seeking to strengthen your selection of CAI teams; or a researcher curious about understanding why a client, who, when gently petting a therapy dog, might look up with tear-filled eyes and say "thank you."

References

Crossman, M. K. (2017). Effects of interactions with animals on human psychological distress. *Journal of Clinical Psychology, 73*, 761–784. doi: 10.1002/jclp.22410.

Crossman, M. K., Kazdin, A. E., Matijczak, A., Kitt, E. R., & Santos, L. R. (2018). The influence of interactions with dogs on affect, anxiety, and arousal in children. *Journal of Clinical Child & Adolescent Psychology*. Early online publication. doi: 10.1080/15374416.2018.1520119.

Griffin, J. A., McCune, S., Maholmes, V., & Hurley, K. (2011). Human-animal interaction research: An introduction to issues and topics. In P. McCardle, S. McCune, J. A. Griffin, & V. Maholmes (Eds.), *How animals affect us: Examining the influence of human-animal interaction on child development and human health* (pp. 3–9). Washington, DC: American Psychological Association.

GuideStar. (2018). About us. Retrieved December 29, 2018, from https://learn.guide star.org/about-us

Herzog, H. (2011). The impact of pets on human health and psychological well-being: Fact, fiction, or hypothesis? *Current Directions in Psychological Science, 20*, 236–239. doi: 10.1 177/0963721411415220.

Herzog, H. (2014). Does animal-assisted therapy really work?: What clinical trials reveal about the effectiveness of four-legged therapists [online]. *Psychology Today*. Retrieved from www.psychologytoday.com/blog/animals-and-us/201411/does-animal-assisted-therapy-really-work [accessed 26 November 2016].

Marino, L. (2012). Construct validity of animal-assisted therapy and activities: How important is the animal in AAT? *Anthrozoos, 25*, 139–151. doi: 10.1016/S0887-6158(02)00199-8.

Ng, Z., Albright, J., Fine, A. H., & Peralta, J. (2015). Our ethical and moral responsibility: Ensuring the welfare of therapy animals. In A. H. Fine (Ed.), *Handbook on animal-assisted therapy: Foundations and guidelines for animal-assisted interventions* (pp. 357–376). New York: Elsevier.

Appendix A

Canine-Assisted Intervention Team Screening Form

Basic Information

Handler	Dog
Name: _____	Dog name: _____
Address: _____	Date of birth *or* Age: _____
_____	Breed: (*e.g., poodle, mixed breed*)
Phone number: _____	_____
E-mail address: _____	Spayed/Neutered? Yes ☐ No ☐
Date of Birth: _____	

Motivation to Volunteer

Handler	Dog
What motivates you to volunteer with your dog with this organization?	What makes you think your dog would enjoy working with [this population]?
_____	_____
_____	_____
How do you think you and your dog could make an impact on the population we serve?	How does your dog respond when she or he is around [this population]?
_____	_____
_____	_____
_____	_____

Relationship

Handler	Dog
How would you describe your dog?	How would your dog describe you?
_____	_____
What makes you think that you and your dog would make a good team?	How long has your dog lived with you?
_____	Where did you acquire your dog?
_____	_____

Temperament

Handler	*Dog*
Describe how you meet new people.	How does your dog behave when she/he is introduced to strangers?
	Many dogs respond differently to various types of people. Describe how your dog responds to:
What would you talk about or do if you met a person, such as a person who wanted to pet your dog, for the first time?	☐ Children: _____ ☐ Women: _____ ☐ Men: Seniors: _____ ☐ People with beards: _____ ☐ People with hats: _____
	☐ People with different skin colors:
	☐ People using crutches or walkers:
	☐ People in wheelchairs:

Experience

Handler	*Dog*
List previous volunteer experience and dates served at each organization (e.g., volunteer organizations and dates).	List any relevant volunteer experience for the dog (e.g., Pet Partners).
Describe your current employment, if applicable (employer, position, and dates).	Has your dog ever served in the following ways? (Check all that apply.) ☐ Emotional support animal ☐ Service dog ☐ Assistance dog (e.g., guide dog) ☐ Facility dog ☐ Military dog ☐ Police dog ☐ Other

Experience With Animals

Handler	Dog
Describe positive experiences you've had with animals.	Describe positive experiences your dog has had with humans and other animals.
Describe any negative experiences you've had with animals.	Describe any negative experiences your dog has had with humans or other animals.

Training

Handler	Dog

Have you and/or your dog participated in dog training?
Yes ☐   No ☐

If yes, what type of training? (Check all that apply.)

- ☐ Puppy
- ☐ Intermediate
- ☐ Advanced
- ☐ Agility
- ☐ Tricks
- ☐ E-collar
- ☐ Board and train
- ☐ Therapy dog
- ☐ Assistance dog (e.g., guide dog)
- ☐ Service dog
- ☐ Facility dog
- ☐ Military or police work

Training facility: _____
Trainer name and credentials: _____
Have you and your dog earned any registrations or certifications (e.g., Canine Good Citizen)
Yes ☐   No ☐
If yes, please list: _____

Background Check

Handler	Dog
As part of working with our organization, we require a background check. Please complete the attached background check form.	Growling is a way that dogs warn others that they feel anxious or threatened. Describe occasions when you have heard your dog growl.

Handler	Dog
	Dogs may lunge, snap, or bite when they feel vulnerable or in danger. Describe any occasions in which your dog has lunged at, snapped at, or bitten a person or animal.

Equipment

Handler	Dog

What type of collar have you used for daily use or training? (Check all that apply.)

☐ Standard nylon/leather neck collar
☐ Martingale
☐ Choke
☐ Prong
☐ Electric or e-collar
☐ Shock collar
☐ Gentle leader
☐ Halter
☐ Other (*please specify*): _____

What type of leash have you used for daily use or training? (Check all that apply.)

☐ Standard nylon/leather leash
☐ Retractable leash
☐ Chain leash
☐ Harness
☐ Seat belt/safety leash (for car)
☐ Other (*please specify*): _____

Describe any equipment needed for you to serve as a therapy dog team.

Describe any equipment needed for your dog to serve as a therapy dog team.

Availability

Handler	Dog

What days and times during the week are you and your dog available to participate in programs?

☐ Sunday Times: _____
☐ Monday Times: _____
☐ Tuesday Times: _____
☐ Wednesday Times: _____
☐ Thursday Times: _____
☐ Friday. Times: _____
☐ Saturday Times: _____

Appendix B
Canine Health Screening Form

Handler's Name: _____

Canine Profile

Name: _____

Date of birth: _____ Age: _____

Breed: _____

Describe dog's temperament: _____

_____

Describe any issues with temperament, anxiety, or aggression: _____

_____

_____

_____

Canine Health

Date of last complete exam: _____

Date of rabies vaccination: _____

Result of annual fecal exam: _____

Result of heartworm exam: _____

Current medications: _____

Describe any conditions or disabilities the dog has and how this may impact therapy work:

_____

_____

_____

_____

Attestations

☐ This dog is current on all vaccinations.
☐ This dog does not display any signs of infectious canine or zoonotic diseases.
☐ This dog is free from internal and external parasites.
☐ I certify that this animal is in good health as of the date of the last complete exam.
☐ I have no reservations about this dog serving as a therapy dog.

Veterinary hospital: _____

Veterinarian name (Print): _____

Veterinarian signature: _____

Date: _____

Appendix C
Canine-Assisted Counseling Skills Checklist

| Date: _____ | CAC team: _____ |
| Client and age: _____ | Observer: _____ |

This form is used to assess a practitioner's canine-assisted counseling skills during a single session.

Ratings: N—Not applicable/No opportunity to observe; O—Does not demonstrate this skill; 1—Demonstrates this skill minimally; 2—Demonstrates this skill variably; 3—Demonstrates this skill consistently

Skill	Skill Description	Rating	Comments
Preliminary Skills			
Appearance and grooming	The practitioner is dressed appropriately for CAC sessions. The dog was bathed and groomed prior to the session.		
Hygiene	The practitioner asks the client to wash hands or use hand sanitizer prior to touching the dog.		
Greeting the dog	The practitioner shows the client how to greet the dog prior to the client meeting the dog. The practitioner guides the greeting interaction between the client and the dog.		
Dog bonding time	The practitioner begins the session with at least 5 minutes of client and dog bonding time.		
Teaching canine communication	The practitioner teaches the client about species-specific canine communication skills during the session.		

(Continued)

(Continued)

Skill	Skill Description	Rating	Comments
Canine welfare	The practitioner ensures that the dog is healthy and well rested, has access to fresh water, and receives a break each hour.		
Facilitative and advanced skills			
Reflection of nonverbal behavior (i.e., tracking)	The practitioner demonstrates reflection of nonverbal behavior in relation to CAC interactions.		
Reflection of content	The practitioner demonstrates reflection of verbal content in relation to CAC interactions.		
Reflection of feeling	The practitioner demonstrates reflection of feeling in relation to CAC interactions.		
Nonverbal skills	The practitioner demonstrates effective use of head, eyes, hands, feet, posture, and voice with the client and dog.		
Empathy	The practitioner communicates empathy, respect, and unconditional positive regard to the client and dog.		
Client-canine relationship	The practitioner demonstrates facilitation of the client-canine relationship so that a working alliance is developed.		
Questions	The practitioner demonstrates appropriate use of open-ended and close-ended questions, with an emphasis on open-ended questions.		
Limit setting	The practitioner sets limits with the client or dog as needed to promote positive human-canine interaction. The practitioner redirects the client or dog immediately when the dog shows stress signals. The practitioner discusses reasons for limit setting or redirection in relation to the human-canine bond.		

Skill	Skill Description	Rating	Comments
Facilitative and advanced skills			
Client-canine communication and response	The practitioner observes the client and dog throughout the session for stress signals. The practitioner responds immediately to reduce client or canine stress and promote safety.		
Canine-specific boundaries	The practitioner ensures that the dog participates in ways that are safe and comfortable for the dog. The dog is allowed to choose to participate or not during the session.		
Confidence	The practitioner demonstrates appropriate levels of self-assurance and trust in her or his own ability and the dog's ability.		
Therapeutic intentionality skills			
Goal setting	The practitioner collaborates with the client to establish realistic and measurable goals that address the presenting problem and integrate the dog and CAC techniques.		
Theory	The practitioner demonstrates understanding and appropriate application of a counseling theory as part of CAC.		
Interventions	The practitioner utilizes and develops CAC interventions that integrate the dog into the therapeutic process.		
Intentionality	The practitioner demonstrates a clear understanding of therapeutic intention using theory and CAC interventions to work toward clinical goals.		

Strengths:

Areas for growth:

Appendix D
Canine-Assisted Intervention Team Assessment

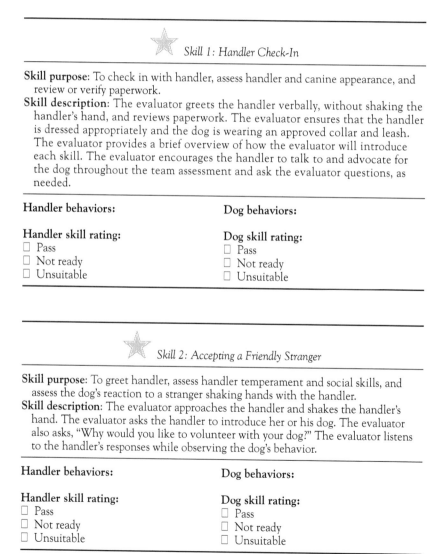

⭐ *Skill 1: Handler Check-In*

Skill purpose: To check in with handler, assess handler and canine appearance, and review or verify paperwork.

Skill description: The evaluator greets the handler verbally, without shaking the handler's hand, and reviews paperwork. The evaluator ensures that the handler is dressed appropriately and the dog is wearing an approved collar and leash. The evaluator provides a brief overview of how the evaluator will introduce each skill. The evaluator encourages the handler to talk to and advocate for the dog throughout the team assessment and ask the evaluator questions, as needed.

Handler behaviors:	**Dog behaviors:**
Handler skill rating:	**Dog skill rating:**
☐ Pass	☐ Pass
☐ Not ready	☐ Not ready
☐ Unsuitable	☐ Unsuitable

⭐ *Skill 2: Accepting a Friendly Stranger*

Skill purpose: To greet handler, assess handler temperament and social skills, and assess the dog's reaction to a stranger shaking hands with the handler.

Skill description: The evaluator approaches the handler and shakes the handler's hand. The evaluator asks the handler to introduce her or his dog. The evaluator also asks, "Why would you like to volunteer with your dog?" The evaluator listens to the handler's responses while observing the dog's behavior.

Handler behaviors:	**Dog behaviors:**
Handler skill rating:	**Dog skill rating:**
☐ Pass	☐ Pass
☐ Not ready	☐ Not ready
☐ Unsuitable	☐ Unsuitable

Skill 3: Teaching How to Greet a Dog

Skill purpose: To assess the handler's ability to teach a person how to greet a dog, assess the handler's ability to advocate for the dog, and assess the dog's interest in interacting with a stranger.

Skill description: The evaluator asks the handler if the evaluator can pet the dog. The handler responds that she or he will teach the evaluator how to greet the dog. The handler then asks the evaluator to approach the dog slowly from the side, stand still (or kneel down and stay still, if the handler has a small dog), and allow the dog to approach and smell the evaluator. When the dog has finished smelling the evaluator, then the handler instructs the evaluator to rub the dog on the chest, back, or other places where the dog likes to be pet. The handler should indicate places where the dog doesn't like to be pet (e.g., "My dog doesn't like being pet on the head or tail, but she really likes getting chest scratches or belly rubs.").

Handler behaviors:	Dog behaviors:
Handler skill rating:	**Dog skill rating:**
☐ Pass	☐ Pass
☐ Not ready	☐ Not ready
☐ Unsuitable	☐ Unsuitable

Skill 4: Sit

Skill purpose: To evaluate how the dog responds to the handler's cue to sit.

Skill description: The evaluator asks the handler to cue the dog to sit. The handler cues the dog to sit. The evaluator then assesses the delivery of the cue by the handler and compliance to this request by the dog.

Handler behaviors:	Dog behaviors:
Handler skill rating:	**Dog skill rating:**
☐ Pass	☐ Pass
☐ Not ready	☐ Not ready
☐ Unsuitable	☐ Unsuitable

Skill 5: Handling

Skill purpose: To assess the dog's overall health and response to being handled.

Skill description: While the dog is in a sitting position, the evaluator looks at the dog's eyes and in the dog's ears and checks all four paws and the dog's nails.

Handler behaviors:	Dog behaviors:
Handler skill rating:	**Dog skill rating:**
☐ Pass	☐ Pass
☐ Not ready	☐ Not ready
☐ Unsuitable	☐ Unsuitable

Skill 6: Down

Skill Purpose: To evaluate how the dog responds to the handler's cue to down.
Skill Description: The evaluator asks the handler to cue the dog to a down position. The handler cues the dog to down. The evaluator then begins to assess handler delivery of the cue and the dog's compliance.

Handler behaviors:	Dog behaviors:

Handler skill rating:	**Dog skill rating:**
☐ Pass	☐ Pass
☐ Not ready	☐ Not ready
☐ Unsuitable	☐ Unsuitable

 Skill 7: Grooming

Skill Purpose: To assess the dog's appearance and grooming.
Skill Description: While the dog is in a down position, the evaluator assesses the dog's appearance by petting the dog's body and tail. The evaluator then takes a soft-bristle brush and brushes the dog's fur three times. The dog's reaction to this is assessed by the evaluator.

Handler behaviors:	Dog behaviors:

Handler skill rating:	**Dog skill rating:**
☐ Pass	☐ Pass
☐ Not ready	☐ Not ready
☐ Unsuitable	☐ Unsuitable

 Skill 8: Walking on a Loose Leash

Skill purpose: To assess how the handler and dog walk together and to ensure the dog can walk calmly next to the handler with a loose leash.
Skill description: *An L-shape that is 10 feet straight ahead and 10 feet to the right will be taped on the floor prior to the assessment.* The evaluator will ask the team to walk on the L-shaped line, making turns as indicated, and turn and walk back when they get to the end of the line. Before the teams starts, the evaluator instructs the team that he or she will stop the team at some point while they are walking. The evaluator will stop the team just after they get to the end of the L, turn around, and start walking back.

Handler behaviors:	Dog behaviors:

Handler skill Rating:	**Dog skill rating:**
☐ Pass	☐ Pass
☐ Not ready	☐ Not ready
☐ Unsuitable	☐ Unsuitable

Skill 9: Walking Through a Crowd

Skill purpose: To assess how teams manage walking through a crowd.

Skill description: The evaluator will ask the team to walk in a straight line toward the back of the room. While the team is walking, a person walking unsteadily with a walker, crutches, or mobility aid will walk in front of the team from the left; another person (walking steadily) will walk in front of the team from the right; and a third person will walk behind the team from the right.

Handler behaviors:	Dog behaviors:
Handler skill rating:	**Dog skill rating:**
☐ Pass	☐ Pass
☐ Not ready	☐ Not ready
☐ Unsuitable	☐ Unsuitable

Skill 10: Managing Several People Who Want to Pet the Dog

Skill purpose: To assess how the handler manages several people who want to pet the dog at the same time.

Skill description: The evaluator tells the handler that the three people approaching want to pet the dog, one of whom is a child and another of whom is in a wheelchair. The handler instructs all three people to space out next to each other, about a foot apart. The handler states that each person will take a turn petting the dog. The handler teaches all three people how to greet the dog (as presented in the *teaching how to greet a dog* skill). The handler then allows the dog to sniff and greet each person. The handler will bring the dog next to the person in the wheelchair or pick the dog up, if the dog is a small dog.

Handler behaviors:	Dog behaviors:
Handler skill rating:	**Dog skill rating:**
☐ Pass	☐ Pass
☐ Not ready	☐ Not ready
☐ Unsuitable	☐ Unsuitable

Skill 11: Reaction to Distractions

Skill purpose: To assess how the team responds to distractions while walking.

Skill description: The evaluator will ask the team to walk in a straight line toward the front of the room. While the team is walking, a person will jog by in front of the team from the left and a person in the back of the room will start a vacuum for three seconds (this sound should be consistent across all team assessments).

Handler behaviors:	Dog behaviors:
Handler skill rating:	**Dog skill rating:**
☐ Pass	☐ Pass
☐ Not ready	☐ Not ready
☐ Unsuitable	☐ Unsuitable

Skill 12: Reaction to a Team With a Neutral Dog

Skill purpose: To assess how the team responds to a neutral dog.

Skill description: The evaluator will ask the team to walk to the opposite end of the room and invite a neutral dog team to enter the room. Both dogs should be placed on the outside (e.g., if a dog walks on the left side of the handler, both dogs would walk on the left side of their handlers and the handlers would walk toward each other, so the handlers are passing each other). The evaluator asks both teams to walk toward each other and directs the handlers to stop next to each other, shake hands, and briefly greet each other. The dog in the team being assessed should not cross in front of the handler to interact with either member of the neutral dog team when the handlers pause to greet each other. The evaluator will direct both teams to continue walking after the brief greeting. The neutral dog team should leave the room right after this skill is completed.

Handler behaviors:	Dog behaviors:
Handler skill rating:	**Dog skill rating:**
☐ Pass	☐ Pass
☐ Not ready	☐ Not ready
☐ Unsuitable	☐ Unsuitable

Skill 13: Stay

Skill purpose: To assess how the dog responds to the handler's cue to stay.

Skill description: The evaluator asks the handler to hold onto their leash, attach the long leash, then hold onto the long leash, and take the original leash off. The evaluator asks the handler to cue the dog to a sit or down position, and then cue the dog to stay. The evaluator then asks the handler to face away from the dog, walk 10 feet away, then turn around and face the dog. The evaluator then asks the handler to pause for 3 seconds, then walk back to the dog.

Handler behaviors:	Dog behaviors:
Handler skill Rating:	**Dog skill rating:**
☐ Pass	☐ Pass
☐ Not ready	☐ Not ready
☐ Unsuitable	☐ Unsuitable

Skill 14: Come When Called

Skill purpose: To assess how the dog responds to the handler's cue to come when called.

Skill description: The dog should stay in a sit or down position from the previous skill. The evaluator asks the handler to cue the dog to stay. The evaluator then asks the handler to face away from the dog, walk 10 feet away, then turn around and face the dog. The evaluator then asks the handler to pause for 3 seconds, then cue the dog to come.

⭐ *Skill 14: Come When Called*

Handler behaviors:	Dog behaviors:
Handler skill rating:	**Dog skill rating:**
☐ Pass	☐ Pass
☐ Not ready	☐ Not ready
☐ Unsuitable	☐ Unsuitable

⭐ *Skill 15: Setting a Limit—Restraining Hug*

Skill purpose: To assess how the handler sets limits with a person who wants to hug the dog.

Skill description: The evaluator and handler sit down on the floor with the dog. The evaluator tells the handler that she or he is going to pretend to start the hug the dog and that the handler needs to interrupt and demonstrate the ACT model to set a limit with the evaluator. The evaluator then states, "I'd really like to pet your dog" and starts to reach for the dog to hug the dog. The handler should put her or his hand out to prevent the evaluator from hugging the dog and use wording similar to ACT wording to set limits with the evaluator.

Handler behaviors:	Dog behaviors:
Handler skill rating:	**Dog skill rating:**
☐ Pass	☐ Pass
☐ Not ready	☐ Not ready
☐ Unsuitable	☐ Unsuitable

⭐ *Skill 16: Setting a Limit—Request to Take the Dog*

Skill purpose: To assess how the handler sets limits with a person who wants to take the dog with him or her and away from the handler.

Skill description: The evaluator tells the handler that she or he is going to pretend to be a volunteer coordinator who would like to take the dog to meet some staff members in a staff-only area. The evaluator tells the handler to demonstrate the ACT model with this request. The evaluator then states, "Could I take your dog with me for a few minutes to meet the staff?" and starts to reach for the dog's leash. The handler should put her or his hand out to prevent the evaluator from taking the leash and use wording similar to the ACT wording to set limits with the evaluator (e.g., "I can tell that you'd like to take my dog with you to meet the staff, but my dog has to stay with me at all times because we're a team. My dog and I can come with you into the staff area, or you can bring the staff out here to meet us.").

Handler behaviors:	Dog behaviors:
Handler skill rating:	**Dog skill rating:**
☐ Pass	☐ Pass
☐ Not ready	☐ Not ready
☐ Unsuitable	☐ Unsuitable

Skill 17: Leave It

Skill purpose: To assess how the dog responds when the dog is presented with an opportunity to eat something on the floor and is not allowed to eat it.

Skill description: The evaluator asks the team to walk past a bowl with a treat in it on the ground. The handler can cue the dog to "leave it" once. The dog is not allowed to lick or eat the treat.

Handler behaviors:

Dog behaviors:

Handler skill rating:
- ☐ Pass
- ☐ Not ready
- ☐ Unsuitable

Dog skill rating:
- ☐ Pass
- ☐ Not ready
- ☐ Unsuitable

Skill 18: Accepting a Treat (Optional)

Skill purpose: To assess how the handler guides a person in offering a treat and to assess how the dog responds in accepting a treat.

Skill description: The evaluator asks the handler if she or he can give the dog a treat. The handler instructs the evaluator on how to give a treat (e.g., use a flat or cupped hand, put fingers together, put treat in center of hand, ask dog to sit, and lower hand to under the dog's mouth so the dog can take the treat). The dog should gently take the treat from the evaluator's hand.

Handler behaviors:

Dog behaviors:

Handler skill rating:
- ☐ Pass
- ☐ Not ready
- ☐ Unsuitable

Dog skill rating:
- ☐ Pass
- ☐ Not ready
- ☐ Unsuitable

Overall team strengths:

_____
_____
_____
_____
_____
_____
_____

Overall team areas for growth:

_____
_____
_____
_____
_____
_____
_____

Final team rating:
- ☐ Pass
- ☐ Not ready
- ☐ Unsuitable

Index

Note: Numbers **bold** indicate a table and page numbers and numbers in *italic* indicate a figure on the corresponding page

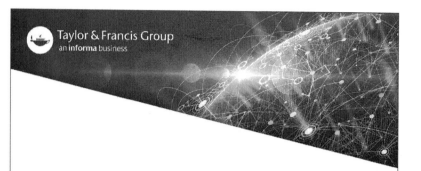